A Primer of
Immunology

F. A. Ward, L.R.C.P.I., M.C. Path.

*Senior Pathologist, Medical School, University
of Natal; Consultant, Natal Institute for Immunology; Formerly Deputy Medical Director,
Natal Blood Transfusion Service; Pathologist,
South African Institute for Medical Research*

London : Butterworths

ENGLAND:	BUTTERWORTH & CO. (PUBLISHERS) LTD. LONDON: 88 Kingsway, WC2B 6AB
AUSTRALIA:	BUTTERWORTH & CO. (AUSTRALIA) LTD. SYDNEY: 20 Loftus Street MELBOURNE: 343 Little Collins Street BRISBANE: 240 Queen Street
CANADA:	BUTTERWORTH & CO. (CANADA) LTD. TORONTO: 14 Curity Avenue, 374
NEW ZEALAND:	BUTTERWORTH & CO. (NEW ZEALAND) LTD. WELLINGTON: 49/51 Ballance Street AUCKLAND: 35 High Street
SOUTH AFRICA	BUTTERWORTH & CO. (SOUTH AFRICA) LTD. DURBAN: 33/35 Beach Grove

Suggested U.D.C. Number: 616–097
Suggested Additional Numbers: 612.017.1
576.8.097

ISBN: 0 407 62570 4

Printed in Great Britain by
Western Printing Services Ltd., Bristol

282071

Contents

Preface

Immunology is a forest of facts and a fair number of fables. Neither makes it easy for the beginner to learn the subject. In this book, therefore, I have tried to lead the reader through the forest by the easiest route while, at the same time, avoiding the fables. It is not intended to be anything like a comprehensive work but, as its name indicates, a Primer.

This approach called for a great deal of selection and in this I was guided by the practical requirements of Medical Students and Medical Practitioners. I hope, nevertheless, that it will prove helpful to Medical Technologists, Nurses and others concerned directly or indirectly with the subject.

The scope and arrangement of the book is such that an index is not necessary. Instead, as in my Primer of Pathology, I give a list of questions at the end with which the reader can test, not only his knowledge, but also the effectiveness of his reading.

It gives me pleasure to record my thanks to Miss June Gordon who prepared most of the diagrams, to Mrs Turkington, who typed the manuscript, and to the Staff of Butterworths, not only for their unfailing courtesy but also for their help in matters too numerous to mention. Finally, I wish to thank the Society of Authors for permission to use an extract from the preface to Bernard Shaw's play, *The Doctor's Dilemma*.

F. A. WARD

Introduction

No one knows how, when, or where it all began. Probably, long before recorded history it was observed that people who survived attacks of certain diseases were not liable to contract these diseases again. Smallpox, manifesting itself through the skin for all to see, being often a fatal disease, and leaving its mark in the form of pock-scars on those fortunate enough to survive, must have been well known even in primitive times. Furthermore, it must have been noticed that those with the scars of previous infection were insusceptible to further attacks. This surely was the first immunological observation.

Passing now from speculation to fact, it was known that variolation was practised in Constantinople in the 18th Century. At this time Constantinople was a busy, bustling city. Situated at the kissing point of two great land masses, it attracted commerce and culture from far and wide. It was here, in the 18th Century, that Lady Mary Wortley Montague, the wife of the British ambassador in Turkey, saw variolation being practised and had the procedure applied to her own son. Subsequently she introduced this rather disgusting and dangerous practice to England where it was accepted because of the widespread incidence of smallpox which it promised to eradicate.

Farmer Jesty and Dr Jenner

A refinement was brought to the problem by a farmer, Jesty, who inoculated his wife with material obtained from a cow suffering from cowpox. Dr Edward Jenner, continuing on this line of thought, eventually published his thesis *An Enquiry into the Causes and Effects of Variola Vacciniae*. That was the beginning of Jennerian vaccination and of Jenner's rise to fame. Significant passages from this famous paper may be quoted at this point—'. . . but what makes cowpox virus so extremely singular is that the person who has been thus affected is forever more after secure from the infection of the smallpox.' That, more or less, sums up his argument. Reporting his second case in this paper, that of a servant girl, who 27 years previously had contracted cowpox, Jenner says, 'In the year 1792, conceiving herself, from this circumstance, secure from the infection of the smallpox, she nursed one of her own children who had already caught the disease, but no indisposition ensued.' From this and from the observations of Jesty, we may reasonably surmise that the principle which made Jenner famous was common knowledge among the local inhabitants. It is therefore strange that Lady Mary's contribution was accepted.

Louis Pasteur

It will be recalled that at this time, although the principle of contagion was known, bacteria and viruses were unknown. Hence, further advances were delayed until the arrival of bacteriology and especially until the arrival of Louis Pasteur. Pasteur was born in 1822, the year before Jenner died. Among many other achievements, he recognized that a virulent organism could become attenuated and that this attenuated organism still maintained its immunological capability. This discovery, now tacitly accepted, was, in fact, a tremendous advance. Attenuation could be brought about by different means, by culturing on artificial media, by passage through a laboratory animal, and, in the example of rabies, by drying the organism. His most celebrated case was that of Joseph Meister, a boy who was severely savaged by a rabid dog. Describing this event Pasteur wrote: 'The death of this child appearing to be inevitable; I decided, not without lively and sore anxiety, as may well be believed, to try upon Joseph Meister the method which I had found constantly successful with dogs. . . .' The boy lived and subsequently became gateman at the Pasteur Institute in Paris.

Salmon and Smith

But even though it was a great advance, the use of attenuated organisms carried an inherent risk; the organism might revert to its original virulent form. This difficulty was resolved, in part at least, by the observations of Salmon and Theobald Smith, who showed that heat-killed organisms still retained their immunological potentiality.

Roux and Yersin

Despite the validity of these discoveries, the nature of immunity remained unknown. The next step in our knowledge was made by Roux and Yersin who discovered, not only the toxin of diphtheria, but that injection of the toxin into a laboratory animal resulted in the appearance of a neutralizing substance in the blood of the injected animal. This neutralizing substance was called antitoxin. Thus the idea grew that when the body was invaded by micro-organisms, it would produce antibodies which served to neutralize the effect, not only of the currently invading organisms but of future invading organisms of the same type. Furthermore it was shown that antitoxin could be taken from one animal and injected into another thereby conferring passive immunity on the second animal. This principle found its greatest application in the prevention and treatment of diphtheria.

Metchnikoff

We must now retrace our steps to follow along a different line of thought which was introduced by the Russian genius Elie Metchnikoff. Metchnikoff was born in 1849, appointed Professor in 1870, Director of the Pasteur Institute in 1895, won the Nobel prize with Paul Ehrlich in 1908 and died in 1916. The following brief bibliography attests the variety and inclinations of his interests,

The Nature of Man (1903)
Old Age (1904)
Immunity to Infectious Diseases (1905)
Some Observations on Soured Milk (1906)

And all this was subsequent to his preparation of anti-lymphocytic serum which he described in 1899 (*Ann. inst. Pasteur*, 1899, **13**, 737).

He will be remembered mainly, however, for his researches in phagocytosis which he began in 1882. 'I was observing', he tells us, 'the life in the mobile cells of a transparent starfish larva, when a new thought suddenly flashed across my brain. It struck me that similar cells might serve in the defence of the organism against intruders.' Thus was conceived the cellular theory of immunity which Metchnikoff championed for the remainder of his life.

Sir Almroth Wright

Metchnikoff had his followers. In this way two factions arose, one claiming humeral factors (antibodies) as the means of bodily immunity and the other claiming cellular factors (phagocytosis). The battle continued for many a year. A sort of peace was brought by the English immunologist, Sir Almroth Wright, who reconciled the two views by introducing his own idea of opsonin. The antibodies, he postulated, enhanced the action of the phagocytes by 'preparing the invaders for phagocytic attack'. Or, to use a metaphor in common use at that time, the opsonin was a sauce which rendered the bacteria more acceptable to the phagocytes.

Charles Richet

These were the really exciting days of immunology. The work of Pasteur and Metchnikoff gave tremendous impetus to further study; more and more research workers became interested and involved. The whole idea of immunity was acceptable not only to doctors but also to the laity, its promise—namely, the eradication of disease—was great and its application seemed financially trivial. Enthusiasm was unrestrained. Those who did not fall in with the general idea were considered backward or reactionary. Such was the temper of the early days of the present century. But even in these early enthusiastic days a few discoveries were made which could not be accommodated in the general notion that immunity was protective in nature. Richet and Smith had shown that in certain instances, repeated antigenic stimulation, far from protecting the animal, actually killed it. This is what Richet called anaphylaxis. But in those days anaphylaxis was a phenomenon seen almost exclusively in laboratory animals; it rarely occurred in Man, so it did not excite much attention.

Bernard Shaw

One man in particular was unmoved by the scene and that was George Bernard Shaw. The following extract is taken from his preface to *The Doctor's Dilemma*, a play of the period from which Sir Almroth Wright fled in disgust. 'On me therefore, the results published by the Pasteur Institute produced no such effect as they did on the ordinary man who thinks that the bite of a mad dog means certain hydrophobia. It seemed to me that the proportion of deaths among the cases treated at the Institute was rather higher, if anything, than might have been expected had there been no Institute in existence.' But Shaw's voice had little influence; vaccination clinics popped up all over the place.

Then two lines of thought began to converge. Long before the disturbing discoveries of Richet (anaphylaxis) and Schick (serum sickness) it was known that certain people reacted in an untoward manner when exposed to pollen, animal dander, certain foodstuffs and indeed a great variety of other substances. The association between these otherwise harmless substances, and the reaction they produced in certain people, was a mystery. Gradually it came to be realized that the association was indeed one of cause and effect and that its basis was immunological. Thus it was seen that immunity was a double edged sword; not only did it prevent disease, it also caused disease. This was a bitter pill to swallow, but worse and still worse was to follow in the form of iso- and auto-immunity.

von Pirquet

Even in these early days there was confusion of language which led to confusion of thought. Facts were accumulating so quickly that they could not be accommodated into a harmonious whole. And in those days harmony was considered almost a *sine qua non* of a scientific thesis. Then suddenly a man of genius called von Pirquet appeared on the scene. He sought to resolve much of the problem by coining a new word, allergy, to convey the idea of changed reactivity. Look at the history of that word. From its original connotation it has, on the one hand, been demoted to refer to some (but not all) instances of changed reactivity, and on the other, it has been extended to such a degree that it has lost all meaning. This topic will be considered at some length in Chapter 10.

Landsteiner and Wiener

A new era and a new department in immunology was opened by Landsteiner at the turn of the century when he discovered the ABO blood group system. The application of this discovery made blood transfusion a feasible, if not completely safe, procedure. This was followed by the discovery of a number of blood group systems of relatively little clinical importance and then, in 1939, in collaboration with Alexander Wiener, he discovered what history may decide is the greatest of all discoveries in this field, the rhesus factor. The application of this discovery not only made blood transfusion the safe procedure that it is today, it led to an understanding of the pathogenesis, then to a rational treatment, and finally to a means of preventing haemolytic disease of the newborn. Further strides in this direction led to the discovery of a great many more blood factors which are now accommodated in some 14 blood group systems.

Antibiotics

In the meantime World War II broke out. Experience in World War I indicated the need for intensive vaccination programmes. Troops were vaccinated against tetanus, typhoid and typhus but there was no vaccine for staphylococci. Prontasil and other sulphonamides, discovered some years earlier, were effective against pneumococci and streptococci, two organisms which rather defied immunological attack, but staphylococci stood unmolested. At this point, British scientists, recalling a discovery made 20 years previously by Fleming, took up the problem and eventually produced penicillin which turned out to be the wonder drug of the late 1940s. So great was the success of penicillin that it stimulated the search for other antibiotics. The search was fruitful and then gradually immunology began to fade into the background. Its promise had not been kept; the freedom from infection enjoyed in those days was due largely to the antibiotics and DDT.

Re-awakening

With the passing of time, however, and it wasn't a very long time, organisms began to develop resistance to penicillin and other antibiotics. Furthermore, penicillin, the most widely used of all the antibiotics, began to produce serious, even fatal, reactions. This was a serious setback. The teeth, as it were, of the antibiotics were being drawn. Then other diseases, against which antibiotics had no effect, were beginning to be seen to have an immunological basis. It seemed that the immunological processes could be directed not only against intruders, but against one's self. All this led to a general awakening of the science of immunology. Further impetus was added by the requirements of organ transplantation, the surgical difficulties of which had been reasonably solved, more and more workers entered the field, more and more papers were published. That is the situation of immunology at the present time.

1—Antigens

Antigens are substances which when injected into an animal stimulate an immunological response in that animal. Several points about this definition need to be considered.

(1) It will be noted that antigens are defined in terms of what they do, not in terms of what they are. In fact, antigens are usually proteins but some very powerful carbohydrate antigens are also known.

(2) The nature of the 'immunological response' is not stated in the definition. The best-known immunological response is the formation of antibodies. Indeed, for many years this was the basis of the standard definition of an antigen—namely, a substance which, when injected into an animal, stimulates the production of antibodies in that animal. In some cases, however, the most prominent immunological response takes the form, not of antibody production, but of delayed hypersensitivity (Chapter 9).

(3) Not mentioned or even implied in the definition are the qualities or attributes which give antigenicity to a substance. The most important of these are as follows.

(a) Foreignness. This means that for a substance to be antigenic it must contain chemical groupings or configurations which are foreign to the host animal.

(b) Molecular weight. All antigens have a large molecular weight. With few exceptions the molecular weight is greater than 5,000 and in some instances it reaches to 1,000,000. This is understandable. A large molecular weight implies a large molecule and a large molecule implies a greater variety in surface configuration and, thus, a greater possibility of foreignness.

1

ANTIGENIC ACTIVITY

Apart from the fundamental attributes of antigens, antigenic activity is dependent on a number of extraneous factors.

Host animal

In any consideration of antigen activity, the animal into which the antigen is injected must be taken into account. Thus, the rhesus antigen (Rh_0) is fairly highly antigenic in Man, but the same antigen is poorly antigenic in rabbits. All rhesus diagnostic antisera are therefore obtained from human sources. Conversely, the blood group antigens M and N are poorly antigenic in Man but they are highly antigenic in rabbits. All M and N diagnostic antisera are therefore obtained from animal (usually rabbit) sources.

Number of antigenic stimulations

The more often a person is stimulated with an antigen the more likely he is to develop an immunological response. It has been shown, for example, that the more often a woman is stimulated by the rehesus antigen the more likely she is to produce rhesus antibodies.

Antigenic exposure during foetal life

Medawar and his associates have shown that an animal would not respond to an antigen if, during foetal life, it had been exposed to that antigen. In other words, for such animals the antigen is, paradoxically, not antigenic. This concept finds practical expression in chimeras. A chimera is an individual who has tissues of another individual living in his body. Chimerism is now well known in human beings in connection with blood groups. Owing to the mixing of the blood of one twin with that of another twin during foetal life, a situation may arise in which one twin possesses two different kinds of blood, his own and his brother's. He may, for example, possess group O red cells (his own) together with group A red cells (his brother's). In this event he would not produce anti-A, an antibody which is universally present in normal group O persons. He would, however, produce anti-B in the normal way. Such a chimera provides a telling example of immunological tolerance acquired *in utero*.

Antigenic specificity

Antigenic specificity is the aspect of antigenic activity which has received most attention. It is commonly and erroneously believed that each antigen stimulates its own single specific antibody. In fact, when an antigen is injected into an animal it stimulates the production not of just one, but of a whole family of antibodies of related specificities (Chapter 2). We can conclude from this observation that a single antigen molecule possesses multiple determinant sites. This is understandable when we recall the enormous size and complex configuration of antigen molecules.

EXAMPLES OF ANTIGENS

Toxins

Toxins are the highly poisonous proteins elaborated by certain bacteria. In addition to being poisonous they are antigenic, but because they are poisonous, they cannot be used as antigens in Man unless they are treated with formaldehyde which converts them into toxoids. Toxoids are non-toxic but they retain the antigenic properties of the toxin from which they were derived. The most common toxoids are those prepared from diphtheria and tetanus bacilli.

Capsules of pneumococci

The polysaccharides of the capsules of pneumococci are the best-known carbohydrate antigens. By means of antibodies prepared against these polysaccharides, the various pneumococci are specifically typed.

A and B iso-antigens

The A and B iso-antigens are also carbohydrate (mucopolysaccharide) antigens and by means of their corresponding antibodies, anti-A and anti-B, the four main blood groups are determined. Witebsky substance is the name given to A and B blood group substance. It is sometimes added to group O blood (to neutralize the anti-A and anti-B) before such blood is given to a group A, B, or AB patient. A and B blood group substance occurs both on the red cells and in the corresponding plasma and secretions as well.

Forssman antigens

Forssman discovered antigens which are similar to one another, but found in a wide variety of animal species. Such antigens are called Forssman antigens. The most notable was his discovery that an antigen in guinea-pig kidney would, in a rabbit, stimulate antibodies reactive against sheep red cells. Similarly, horse serum possesses an

3

A-like antigen as is shown by the fact that an injection of horse serum into a human being (of blood group O) results in a great increase in the titre of anti-A.

Domestic antigens

This term is used here to refer to the antigens (various tissue proteins) present in one's own body. Being domestic (that is, not foreign) they do not generally illicit an immunological response in their natural environment, but on transfer to another human being they evoke a response. That the body does not react against its own tissue antigens is the famous generalization of Ehrlich which he called *horror autotoxicus*. Unfortunately, there are many exceptions to this general rule (Chapter 14).

Tolerance of domestic antigens

Tolerance of domestic antigens is so universal that it is usually tacitly accepted. Yet when one comes to realize that the human body must contain thousands of different protein molecules, all of which are antigenic for other animals, one is led to enquire into the nature of this immunological tolerance.

From the observations on chimeras and the experiments of Medawar we deduce that up to a certain point in foetal life the individual does not recognize foreign proteins immunologically. He seems to accept them as his own. Furthermore, on stimulation with the same antigen after birth, he still does not recognize them. This applies to foreign proteins and to domestic proteins as well. Immunological tolerance to domestic antigens is therefore seen as a phenomenon resulting from exposure of the domestic antigens to the antibody-producing apparatus *in utero* and before the critical point of Medawar. But of the precise mechanism of this phenomenon, we can only speculate.

Haptens

As stated above, one of the physical criteria or conditions for antigenicity is that the antigen molecule be a large molecule. Many small molecular substances, however, can be made antigenic by conjugating them with a protein which functions as a carrier. Such small molecular substances are called haptens. Examples include picric acid, tartaric acid, p-aminobenzoic acid and those used by Landsteiner in his classic experiments—ortho, meta, and para aminosulphonic acid.

Australian antigen

In 1965, Blumberg and his colleagues discovered a mysterious antigen in the serum of an Australian aborigine which is now known as the Australian antigen. Its great interest lies in the fact that it is associated with, and may be identical with, the virus of infective hepatitis. It occurs in about 0·1 per cent of the North American and European population and is demonstrated by an immunodiffusion technique (Chapter 5).

Adjuvants

Adjuvants are substances which, when mixed with antigens, enhance the antigenic activity. The best known are Freund's adjuvant (prepared in two forms, complete and incomplete and used largely in experimental work) and alum, commonly incorporated in preparations of diphtheria toxoid.

2—Antibodies

Antibodies are substances which appear in the serum of an animal in response to antigenic stimulation. It is true that newborn babies, without antigenic stimulation, have antibodies in their sera but these represent a passive transfer of antibodies across the placenta from the mother. In all other normal circumstances antibodies arise from antigenic stimulation.

The presence of antibodies in a serum is revealed by their ability to react *in vitro* with their corresponding antigens. Thus, if a serum reacts with antigen X, we say that it contains antibodies which we call anti-X. The kind of reaction which occurs when antigen and antibody come into contact varies—sometimes a precipitate forms, sometimes agglutination occurs, sometimes complement is fixed. The antibodies are thus often called precipitins, agglutinins, or complement fixing antibodies.

ANALYSIS OF ANTIBODIES

Nature of antibodies

For a long time it has been known that the antibody activity of antisera resided in the protein fraction of the serum. Then the activity was localized to that fraction of the proteins which was precipitated by means of half-saturation with ammonium sulphate. This is the globulin fraction. The next big step was taken in 1939. Tiselius and Kabat, by means of electrophoresis, separated the serum proteins according to their electrophoretic mobilities and localized the bulk of the antibody activity in the slow-moving fraction—gamma globulin (*Figure 1*).

Gamma globulin, a term often misleadingly used in the singular, was then found to be in fact a heterogeneous collection of proteins

6

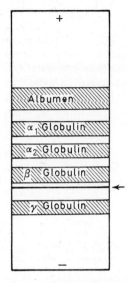

Figure 1 Normal serum electrophoresis. The serum is applied to the strip at the line indicated by the arrow. An electric current is passed through the strip and the different proteins migrate at different rates which depend upon their iso-electric points. The endosmotic flow of the buffer solution, which is in the opposite direction, opposes, to some extent, the movement of the protein molecules. The slow-moving γ globulin molecules move in the opposite direction to the other protein molecules.

of which the fraction now known as Ig G is the most abundant and most important. More recently Ig G itself was found to be a heterogenous mixture and at least four different forms of it have been recognized and named.

But in the meantime antibody activity was detected in globulins other than gamma globulin and before long, with the increasing complexity of things and the increasing complexity of the names of things, confusion fell upon our thought. In 1959, twenty years after Tiselius and Kabat had separated gamma globulin, Heremans proposed that we call all these globulins with antibody activity by the name immunoglobulins or Ig. These will be considered in greater detail in Chapter 4.

Naturally occurring antibodies

The naturally occurring antibodies are antibodies found in the serum of persons who have not had obvious antigenic stimulation. They are, nevertheless, believed to arise from antigenic stimulation during the course of a naturally occurring infection which is often so mild as to pass unnoticed, or as a result of stimulation by a variety of antigens which are present in food, water, and even air. They are usually of low titre but those following infection are of great importance in preventing further attacks by the same type of organism.

Naturally occurring iso-antibodies

Following on Landsteiner's discovery of the ABO blood groups, it soon became apparent that when an antigen is absent from a red cell, the corresponding antibody is present in the serum. These antibodies are commonly referred to as the naturally occurring iso-antibodies or, more precisely, as their characteristic action is agglutination, the naturally occurring iso-agglutinins. The situation in regard to the distribution of these antibodies is shown by the well-known table set out as follows.

TABLE 1

Blood group	Antigen present	Antibody present
A	A	anti-B
B	B	anti-A
AB	A and B	Nil
0	Nil	anti-A and anti-B

This simple and easily remembered statement is sufficient for most purposes, but it leaves some phenomena unexplained. These phenomena will be considered in greater detail in Chapter 11.

Origin of the naturally occurring iso-antibodies

Blood group A and B substances are so widely distributed in nature that contamination with them is inevitable. It is believed, therefore, that the naturally occurring iso-antibodies result from heterogenic stimulation by these antigens.

Antibody specificity

An extraordinary feature of antibody activity is its remarkable specificity. Ehrlich likened this to a lock and key relationship. This, however, is an over-simplification of the case and it gave rise to the false assumption that a single antigen will produce a single specific antibody which will react with it to the exclusion of all else. This is not so. A single antigen, whether it is on a red cell, a bacterial cell, a virus, or whether it is a pure protein antigen, will give rise to a family of antibodies of different but related specificities. This observation leads us to conceive an antigen, even a pure protein antigen, as a composite structure like a string of beads, each bead with a different colour. To extend the analogy, just as this string of beads will cause a variety of optical reactions (because of the different colours of the individual beads) so an antigen will cause a variety of antibodies to appear. This it does by virtue of its possessing a variety of antigenic determinants.

Thus, to return to Ehrlich's analogy, if the antigen is the lock we must accept not only that there are a number of different keys that will open it, but also that there are skeleton keys available too. This will become clearer as we proceed.

Cross reactions

Sometimes it is found that antibodies produced against antigen X will react, not only against X but also against Y. This is an example of a cross reaction. Thus it is found that an antiserum produced against duck globulin will react not only against duck globulin but also against goose globulin. The simplest explanation for this phenomenon is that the duck and goose globulin possess antigenic determinants in common. This is not surprising in two such closely related species.

Are antibody reactions specific?

From what has been said above we can see that antibody reactions are specific but not absolutely specific. This may sound like a contradiction in terms because the word 'specific' is usually thought of as an absolute term. In immunology, however, it is a relative term and as such it functions better if it has an adjective. In the above experiment, for example, the antiserum produced against duck globulin can be made *more* specific by absorbing it with goose globulin. It will then continue to react with duck but not with goose globulin. It might, however, still react with swan globulin; hence further appropriate absorptions will be necessary in order to obtain a *highly* specific antiserum.

Antibodies as antigens

Antibodies, as we have seen, are proteins. It is therefore not surprising that they can act as antigens. Indeed, being globulins, they are very powerful antigens. When they are used as antigens, however, they produce ordinary antiglobulin antibodies just as any other globulin would. It seems, therefore, that the antibody-producing apparatus, while it can distinguish the globulins of various species, cannot distinguish between various antibody specificities. It is important to keep in mind the fact that antibodies are antigenic when we are treating patients with antitoxic serum prepared in, for example, a horse.

9

Antibodies against immunoglobulins

After the immunoglobulins were purified by physical and chemical means it was then possible to use them as antigens. When this was done, highly specific antisera were produced which are now available commercially for the identification of these immunoglobulins.

Gamma globulin groups—allotypes

Formerly it was thought that gamma globulin of one species would not be antigenic for another member of that species. More recently this view has had to be changed. Gamma globulin of one rabbit, for example, may indeed be antigenic for another rabbit and this observation culminated in the discovery of a whole series of immunologically distinct gamma globulins in rabbits. These are genetically determined and are called the allotypes.

That a similar state of affairs exists in human beings is shown by the existence of the Gm types of gamma globulin. These were discovered by means of a peculiar antibody (the RA factor) which is found in the serum of patients with rheumatoid arthritis. Like the gamma globulin allotypes in rabbits, these too are genetically determined.

Concept of complete and incomplete antibodies

Many antibodies (for example, the iso-agglutinins) are capable of reacting with, and causing their characteristic effect (in this case red cell agglutination) when they are added to a *saline* suspension of the corresponding red cells. Thus anti-A agglutinates a saline suspension of group A cells. These are called complete antibodies because they are complete in themselves and need nothing else to bring about their characteristic effect. They are 19S and Ig M in type.

Many other antibodies, however (for example, most Rh antibodies), while combining with the corresponding cells in saline medium, do not agglutinate them. If, however, the cells are suspended in a high *protein* medium they will agglutinate. As these antibodies require something more to bring about agglutination, they are called incomplete antibodies. These are 7S, Ig G in type.

Haemolytic antibodies also require another factor (complement) to bring about their characteristic reaction (haemolysis), but these are not included in the term 'incomplete' antibodies.

Concept of warm and cold antibodies

While most antibodies will react through a fairly wide thermal range, some react best or exclusively at low temperatures, while others react best at body temperature. The former are called cold, and the latter warm, antibodies. These terms are usually applied to auto-antibodies.

Concept of auto-antibodies

Originally it was thought that the body would not produce antibodies against its own tissue antigens. This idea is the basis of Ehrlich's theory of *horror autotoxicus*, which, in general, is true, but in many cases fallacious. The body may indeed produce antibodies reactive against its own tissue antigens—indeed it is commonplace in blood banking to find cold auto-antibodies even in health. In abnormal states, such as acquired haemolytic anaemia, it is common to find both cold and warm types of auto-antibody.

Antibody strength—antibody titre

The strength of an antibody is measured by serological titration. Unlike chemical titration, serological titration is done by making serial dilutions, usually doubling dilutions, of the antiserum in a row of test tubes. The corresponding antigen is then added to each test tube. After a period the tubes are examined and the greatest dilution which gives a positive reaction is noted. The reciprocal of this dilution is the titre. Thus, if the greatest dilution in which a positive reaction occurs is 1/256, the titre is 256.

Further consideration of this procedure brings to light two important points.

(1) It explains why titres are reported in peculiar figures, such as 32, 64, 128, 256, 512, 1024 and so on. This, of course, is because of the doubling dilutions but it is likely to give a false impression of precision.

(2) It shows clearly why serological titrations, even in the hands of an expert and careful technologist, must of necessity be grossly inaccurate especially at the high titres. Fancy using a scale graduated in such a progression to measure the width of this page! You would say it was absurd. It is for this reason that a difference between a titre of 512 and 1024 is regarded as insignificant, while the difference between a titre of 8 and 32 is significant.

Function of antibodies

The circumstances in which antibodies (antitoxins) were first discovered naturally led to the conclusion that these bodies represented a munificent gesture on the part of Nature. Nature, in her bounty, it seemed, protected her favoured creatures against attack from her less favoured ones. In other words, antibodies were protective. This idea was in harmony with the temper of those Victorian days and to some extent it has survived to the present day.

This cosy belief was shattered when it was discovered that, far from protecting against disease, some antibodies could actually cause disease. Today, therefore, it is possible to classify antibodies according to their function into *protective* kinds (for example, the antitoxins) and *pathogenic* (for example, rhesus antibodies). Thus, the impartiality of Nature in regard to antibody production and function is underlined. Later we will see that not only antibody production but the immune mechanism, as a whole, possesses this dual Jekyll and Hyde character.

COMPLEMENT

Since the early days of immunology it was known that while fresh antiserum might cause haemolysis of red cells, it lost this capacity if it were left to stand for a few days. The haemolytic activity could also be abolished by heating the antiserum at 56°C for half an hour and it could be restored by the addition of small amounts of *any* fresh serum. From these observations it was concluded that the haemolytic activity of an antiserum depended on two factors, the haemolytic antibody and a heat-labile factor which is present in all fresh sera. This latter is now called complement.

More recently complement was found to consist, not of one substance, but of at least four, which are designated $C'1$, $C'2$, $C'3$ and $C'4$. The titre of the complement as a whole depends upon the titre of the weakest component which in the human being is $C'2$. Mayer and his colleagues have shown that complement activity in antigen-antibody reactions proceeds in three stages. The first stage seems to involve $C'1$ and $C'4$ and requires calcium ions. The second stage involves $C'2$ and requires magnesium ions, while the third stage involves only $C'3$. Further work has shown that with the possible exception of $C'1$, all these factors are heterogeneous.

That complement is used up in certain antigen-antibody reactions has provided a convenient means of proving that an antigen-antibody reaction has, in fact, occurred. This is the principle involved in various complement-fixation tests.

3—Antibody Production

MODE OF ANTIBODY PRODUCTION

Any theory of the mode of antibody production must accommodate all the known facts of this phenomenon. Unfortunately, there is not complete agreement on these facts—when agreement exists there is often a variation in emphasis, and, as time passes, there is often changing emphasis. The side-chain theory of Ehrlich, for example, was obviously meant to accommodate what was, in those days, the most striking feature of antibody activity—namely, its specificity. But his theory otherwise called for too great a draft on the imagination and is now only of historical interest.

Direct template theory

With the growing realization that antibody activity resided in the protein fraction of the plasma, Landsteiner and others saw antibody formation merely as a modification of protein synthesis, a modification brought about by the presence of antigens. According to this view, when an antigen enters the body it is taken up by phagocytic cells. In these cells it serves as a die, or mould, or cast, or template against which globulin synthesis proceeds. Thus, the cell produces molecules with a physical configuration which fits the antigen exactly. These globulin molecules, now called antibodies, are produced in abundance and released into the blood stream.

This theory, which remained popular in one form or another until the late 1940s, was also obviously aimed at explaining antibody specificity to the neglect or exclusion of other facts which had been well established. It did not, for example, explain why antibody production continued after the antigen could be reasonably presumed to have left the body.

13

Indirect template theory

Although the *horror autotoxicus* view of Ehrlich was shown not to be universally valid, it was valid enough to impress Burnet and Fenner who felt that it ought to be accommodated in any theory of antibody production. They also sought to accommodate the neglected fact that antibody formation continued long after the antigen had disappeared. Thus they introduced a view which is now known as the indirect template theory. According to this, domestic antigens carry a mark which identifies them as such to the cells of the antibody-producing apparatus. The mark not only identifies the antigen but also precludes it from the possibility of functioning as an antigen. In this way a rational explanation was given for the reason why the body does not produce antibodies against its own (domestic) antigens.

As for the continuation of antibody production, here is where the spark of genius enters. Burnet and Fenner saw the antigen not only as a mould or cast or template as in the direct template theory, but also as something which, by interfering with the genetic mechanism of the cell, changed its reproductive potentialities. From henceforth not only would the cell produce antibodies, but its daughter cells would do so too. Thus, antibody synthesis would continue. In short, the antigen in effect was, at the same time, a template and a mutogen.

Jerne's theory

Almost 100 years after Darwin published his *Origin of Species by Means of Natural Selection*, Jerne, a Danish immunologist with a remarkable flexibility of mind, published the *Natural Selection Theory of Antibody Formation*. Here was an entirely new approach. Jerne saw in the globulin molecules of the plasma, reactive sites capable of combining with all (except domestic) antigens. This is probably not such an extreme view as it first appears. The antigen, on entering the body, seeks out the globulin with the corresponding reactive sites, combines with it and carries it to the antibody-producing apparatus. There it is replicated over and over again. The theory has the great virtue of originality, but while it solved some problems, it raised others.

Clonal selection theory of Burnet

Sir Macfarlane Burnet, applying himself once more to the problem of antibody production, but now in the light of Jerne's theory, advanced his clonal selection theory. In this he shifts the emphasis

14

from the circulating globulin molecules to surface sites on the cells of the antibody-producing apparatus. The antigen enters the body, seeks out the cells which have the corresponding reactive sites on their surfaces and combines with them. This causes proliferation of the cells. Thus, a clone of cells producing specific antibodies comes into existence.

Lymphocyte receptor theory

Yet another theory of antibody production puts lymphocytes to the forefront. According to this view lymphocytes are endowed with receptors which are capable of recognizing all foreign antigens. As it is generally accepted that only antibodies can recognize antigens these receptors are seen as small samples of antibody fixed on the surface of the lymphocytes. Their formation, like that of other proteins, is determined by de-oxyribonucleic acid (DNA). The lymphocyte, as it courses through the various channels of the body, is exposed to whatever foreign material may be present. If any antigen which it encounters 'fits' its particular receptor, an immune response is initiated, and the lymphocyte undergoes a series of transformations culminating in the formation of a plasma cell which produces the antibodies.

This theory requires an even greater feat of the imagination than the others before it can be seriously entertained. But this alone should not disqualify it. When we think of the undoubted ability of the antibody-producing apparatus to recognize many thousands, perhaps millions, of different antigens (or antigenic determinants) we must conclude that any satisfactory theory of antibody formation must of necessity stagger the imagination.

SITE OF ANTIBODY PRODUCTION

Up until now I have been referring from time to time to the 'antibody-producing apparatus' without saying where this apparatus was located or how it was constituted. Now is the time to consider these things.

Organs

For a long time it has been known that antibodies were formed mainly in the spleen and lymphatic glands. Both these organs have been found, under suitable experimental conditions, to produce antibodies *in vitro*. The spleen seems to be the more important organ when the antigen is given by the intravenous route, and the lymphatic glands when it is given intramuscularly or subcutaneously.

Because the spleen and lymphatic glands produce antibodies, it seems reasonable to believe that antibody production occurs wherever there are accumulations of lymphoid cells. Furthermore, there is evidence to show that antibodies can even be produced locally at the site of antigen injection. This is more likely to occur if the antigen is given with an adjuvant which causes the formation of a granuloma. Such a granuloma might be looked upon as an artificially induced antibody-producing apparatus.

Cells

The cells of lymphoid tissue consist essentially of lymphocytes, plasma cells and macrophages. In the past there has been considerable controversy as to which of these cells are responsible for antibody production. The following observations bear heavily on this question. Antigenic stimulation results in an increase of plasma cells in local lymphatic glands; by the Coons immunofluorescence technique, antibodies have been demonstrated in plasma cells, and finally, in cases of hypogammaglobulinaemia, there is a marked deficiency of both plasma cells and antibodies. There is therefore little doubt that plasma cells, or their immediate precursors, are responsible for at least the final stages of antibody production.

But what about the early stages? The plasma cell is not a phagocyte and it seems to have little direct relationship with antigens. Here is where other cells have to be involved and in this matter there is no general agreement. One thing, however, seems reasonable—while the plasma cell is the last to be involved in antibody production, it looks as though the macrophage, which is a phagocyte, is the first. Indeed there is evidence that antibody formation results from the concerted action of macrophage, lymphocyte and plasma cell.

4—Immunoglobulins

The word immunoglobulin is a collective noun proposed by Heremans to include all the globulins which have antibody activity. It also includes similar proteins which have no such activity.

ANALYSIS OF IMMUNOGLOBULINS

Anatomy of the immunoglobulins

In 1962, Porter and his colleagues, by means of proteolytic enzymes, dissected a molecule of immunoglobulin and found it to consist of a pair of heavy chains and a pair of light chains. These chains are bound together by di-sulphide linkages (*Figure 2*). It is now believed that all immunoglobulins have a similar basic structure.

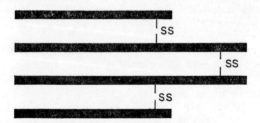

Figure 2 To show the structure of an immunoglobulin molecule. Note the two heavy chains, the two light chains and the disulphide linkages.

The light chains were called kappa and lambda and are symbolized by the Greek letters κ and λ respectively. Five different kinds of heavy chains have so far been discovered and these are called gamma (γ), alpha (α), mu (μ), delta (δ) and epsilon (ϵ).

17

Nomenclature of the immunoglobulins

This general information, if it is known in a particular case, is conveyed in the name of the immunoglobulin. Thus, Ig G refers to an immunoglobulin which has a pair of gamma chains, Ig A refers to an immunoglobulin with a pair of alpha chains, and Ig M refers to one with a pair of mu chains. If, in addition, the identity of the light chains is known, then this information would also be conveyed in the name. Thus, Ig GK would refer to an immunoglobulin with two gamma (heavy) chains and two kappa (light) chains (*Figure 3*).

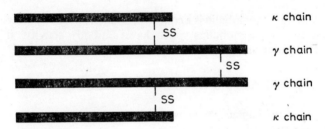

Figure 3 To illustrate the nomenclature of the immuno-globulins; the heavy chains of the immunoglobulins are designated γ, α, μ, δ and ε. The light chains are designated κ and λ. The full name given to a particular immunoglobulin depends on its constituent chains. The above example, containing two γ chains and two κ chains would be called Ig GK and its molecular formula would be $\gamma_2\kappa_2$. In nature, each immunoglobulin molecule is chemically symmetrical, i.e. it has two identical light chains and two identical heavy chains.

An alternative and possibly clearer way of indicating the molecular structure is by using the abbreviated molecular formula. The symbol and the abbreviated molecular formula are given side by side for comparison, as shown below.

Ig GK	$\gamma_2\kappa_2$	Ig GL	$\gamma_2\lambda_2$
Ig AK	$\alpha_2\kappa_2$	Ig AL	$\alpha_2\lambda_2$
Ig MK	$\mu_2\kappa_2$	Ig ML	$\mu_2\lambda_2$

As each naturally occurring immunoglobulin, however, has two identical heavy chains and two identical light chains, all the information required is conveyed by means of the symbol. The molecular formula is therefore redundant for the purpose of identification except in artificially produced immunoglobulins.

Effects of proteolytic enzyme digestion

The anatomy of the immunoglobulin molecule has been explored largely by the use of such proteolytic enzymes as papain and pepsin. These enzymes attack the molecule at different sites, the resulting fragments are then further examined by means of the ultra-centrifuge, electrophoresis, and their antigenic reactions. *Figure 4* shows the effect of papain digestion.

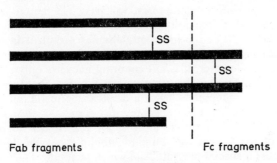

Fab fragments   Fc fragments

Figure 4 The effect of papain digestion.

Papain digestion breaks the immunoglobulin into two kinds of fragments. One kind retains the antibody activity of the original immunoglobulin molecule and is called Fab to remind us of this fact. The other kind of fragment does not possess antibody activity but because it is crystallizable it is called Fc. The broken line indicates the points of papain cleavage. That part of the heavy chain which forms part of the Fab fragment is called the Fd piece.

A comparison between the important immunoglobulins

Although all immunoglobulins have essentially the same basic structure, they differ from each other in several respects. These differences are summarized in Table 2.

TABLE 2

	Ig G	Ig A	Ig M
Sedimentation constant	7S	7–15S	19S
Molecular weight	160,000	400,000	1,000,000
Crosses placenta	Yes	No	No

Capacity to cross the placenta

Whether an immunoglobulin can cross the placenta or not is a point of great practical importance. The naturally occurring iso-agglutinins (anti-A and anti-B) in the mother's blood, being 19S, Ig M immunoglobulins, do not pass to the baby. Some rhesus antibodies are also of the same type and these too do not pass to the baby and are therefore harmless. But more often rhesus antibodies are of the Ig G variety. These readily cross the placenta to cause haemolytic disease in the baby.

Similarly, all other Ig G antibodies which the mother may possess against various infectious diseases, will pass, via the placenta, and thus confer passive immunity on the baby. Such an immunity, possibly against most of the infectious diseases prevalent in the community into which the baby is born, is obviously of great importance. Being passive, however, it is not enduring but lasts only about four to six months. During this time it may interfere with attempts to produce active immunity—hence a case can be made out for postponing vaccination until after six months of age.

The ability of an antibody to cross the placenta is not simply a function of the size of the immunoglobulin molecule. Ig G molecules possess a special placental site which facilitates their passage.

Ig G variants

Further experiments show that Ig G is not a homogeneous protein but a class of proteins consisting of at least four serologically distinct types. These types have been called Ig Ga, Ig Gb, Ig Gc, and Ig Gd. These sub-units have been found to differ in their heavy chains but not in their light chains. $IgG\ 1, 2, 3, 4$

Light chain variants

Bence-Jones proteins are light chains of immunoglobulins which appear to be synthesized in excess in cases of myelomatosis. Instead of being linked with heavy chains, they are excreted in the urine. A Bence-Jones protein in a given patient may differ from that in another patient, but it is always the same in that given patient and it is almost always identical with the light chains of his myeloma proteins. Antisera prepared in rabbits reactive against a given Bence-Jones protein, will react with one or other, but not both light chains. That is to say, they are either anti-K or anti-L corresponding with the κ or the λ chains of the patient's immunoglobulin.

Allotypes

For a long time it has been known that serum from certain persons, especially those suffering from rheumatoid arthritis, contains antibodies which would react against gamma globulin. These antibodies were detected by the fact that they caused agglutination of red cells previously coated with incomplete antibodies. This is the basis of the Rose-Waller test for rheumatoid arthritis. Further investigation of this peculiar phenomenon by Grubb led to the discovery of two markers on the immunoglobulin molecule. These markers are now designated Gm and InV. The Gm markers are on the heavy, and the InV on the light chains. These subgroups of Ig G are distinct from, but nevertheless related to, the subgroups previously described and designated Ig Ga, Ig Gb, Ig Gc, and Ig Gd.

Immunoglobulin G

Immunoglobulin G is the most abundant of the immunoglobulins of the serum; it accounts for more than 85 per cent of the total. It has a molecular weight of about 160,000 and a sedimentation constant of about 7S. Being the most abundant it is natural that it would be the most actively studied of all the immunoglobulins and much of what has been discovered in Ig G has been assumed to apply to the others also. Most of the antibody activity of the serum resides in this immunoglobulin.

Immunoglobulin M

Immunoglobulins of this type have a greater molecular weight (1,000,000) a greater sedimentation constant (19S), and a greater electrophoretic mobility than the others. They are the first to be detected after antigenetic stimulation but they soon disappear to be replaced by the Ig G type. This, however, is not an invariable rule— the naturally occurring iso-antibodies, anti-A and anti-B, are of this type and they persist for life. These immunoglobulins are destroyed by the action of 2-mercaptoethenol and on this fact is based a simple test for distinguishing them from Ig G antibodies of the same specificity. They do not cross the placenta and while they have InV markers on their light chains, they do not have Gm markers on their heavy chains. Recently it has been suggested that some of the bactericidal activity of serum depends on Ig M and that if this immunoglobulin is deficient an infection with meningococci, for example, may be rapidly fatal. The same, it seems, may apply to other Gram negative organisms also. Ig M is reported to be increased in cases of trypanosomiasis and decreased in cases of coeliac disease.

Immunoglobulin A

Immunoglobulins of the A type are much less abundant than Ig G in the serum, but they are much more abundant than Ig G in tears, saliva, the secretions of the nasopharynx and colostrum. These observations suggest that Ig A antibodies have a special role in the protection of the conjunctivae and the upper respiratory tract from infection. It is interesting that there is a custom in certain parts of Italy for a lactating mother to squirt colostrum from her breast into her baby's eyes should they be inflamed. Like Ig M, these immunoglobulins have InV markers on their light chains but no Gm markers on their heavy chains. Low levels of Ig A have been reported in cases of steatorrhoea.

Immunoglobulin D

Immunoglobulins of the D type occur in very small quantities in normal serum; sometimes they cannot even be detected. Antibody activity has not been associated with these immunoglobulins.

Immunoglobulin E

The reagin type of antibodies which cause immediate hypersensitivity in Man, is now regarded as E type immunoglobulin (Ishizaka). This has been shown by using Ig E to block a Prausnitz-Kustner reaction. The antibodies cannot be detected in the serum by conventional methods of serology, but special two-stage procedures have been developed which, though complicated, may be of great value in investigating cases of immediate hypersensitivity in the future.

5—Antigen-Antibody Reactions

LABORATORY ASPECTS

There are two aspects of antigen-antibody reactions to be considered, the clinical and the laboratory aspects. In this chapter we shall deal with the laboratory aspects, the remainder of the book is devoted largely to the clinical aspects.

Antigen-antibody reactions in the laboratory are often plainly visible but in some cases they are completely invisible. In these it is necessary to employ some device to show that a reaction has, in fact, occurred. For this, and other reasons, many different and complicated tests have been devised to demonstrate antigen-antibody reactions. The principle involved in these tests will be discussed here.

Generally, antigen-antibody reactions can be used to identify the antigen, if the antibody is known, and to identify the antibody, if the antigen is known.

Precipitin reactions

Precipitin reactions in one form or another are designed to show the action of precipitating antibodies. In their simplest form the soluble antigen is placed in a narrow bore test tube and onto this a solution of antibodies (usually an antiserum) is layered. At the interface between the two solutions a white line of precipitate forms if an antigen-antibody reaction has taken place.

Ouchterlony technique

Ouchterlony improved the above method by placing the antigen and antibody solutions in small wells cut in agar. Antigen and antibody diffuse towards one another through the agar and where they meet a white line of precipitate forms. The great advantage of this technique is that, should there be multiple antigens in the solution, and should the antiserum contain the corresponding antibodies, then multiple lines of precipitate will appear in the agar. The Ouchterlony

23

technique will also establish the identity, or lack of identity, between antigens and antibodies (*Figures 5 to 7*).

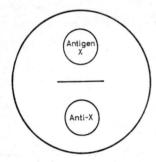

Figure 5 An Ouchterlony preparation in its simplest form. The antigen, in the upper well, and the antibody in the lower, diffuse towards each other and where they meet, a white line of precipitate forms. The precise position and shape of the line depends on the rate of diffusion of the reactants through the agar, and this depends on the concentration and the molecular weight of the reactants. A straight line, half way between the two wells, as in this example, indicates similar concentrations and similar molecular weights.

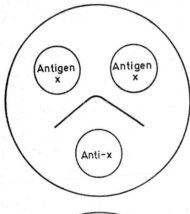

Figure 6 An Ouchterlony preparation showing the reaction of identity. If the same antigen is placed in the upper wells and the corresponding antibody in the lower one, then fusion of the two lines of precipitate, as shown in the diagram, will occur. If the antigen in the upper right-hand well were unknown, and if fusion of the lines of precipitate occurred, then it could be concluded that the unknown antigen was identical to that in the left-hand well.

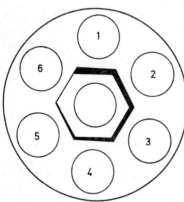

Figure 7 An Ouchterlony titration. The wells numbered 1, 2, 3, 4, 5, and 6, contain increasing dilutions of the antigen solution. The central well contains the corresponding antiserum. The hexagonal line of decreasing thickness represents the antigen-antibody precipitate. It will be seen that even in the greatest dilution there was still a faint reaction.

24

Grabar-Williams technique—immunoelectrophoresis

Grabar and Williams brought a further refinement to the procedure by introducing electrophoresis. In this experiment the antigen solution is placed in a well in the agar and then a current of electricity is passed. The various protein molecules in the solution migrate according to their electrophoretic mobilities. After a period the current is stopped and antiserum is placed in a trough cut in the agar parallel to the line of migration of the protein molecules. Antibodies in the antiserum, and the now separated antigens, diffuse towards one another and where they meet a white line of precipitate forms (*Figure 8*).

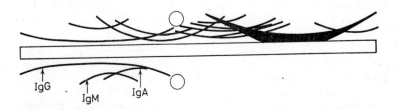

IgG   IgM   IgA

Figure 8 To show immunoelectrophoresis by the Grabar-Williams technique. Human serum was placed in the top well and a mixture of Ig G, Ig A, and Ig M was placed in the bottom well. After electrophoresis, anti-human serum was placed in the trough. The arc lines show the various antigen-antibody precipitates.

Agglutination reactions

In the simplest form of these reactions, particles containing the antigen are mixed with the antiserum, which contains the antibodies. The particles are usually either red cells or bacteria but sometimes inert particles to which an antigen has been artificially attached are used. After a period, the mixture is examined and if the particles are found to be agglutinated, it indicates that an antigen-antibody reaction has occurred.

This reaction is employed in the grouping of red blood cells and bacteria, the antigens being naturally occurring on the cells. For other purposes the red cells may be tanned (with tannic acid) or treated with chromic chloride. In this condition they will absorb extraneous antigens. The subsequent addition of the corresponding antibodies will result in a reaction with this extraneous antigen and the red cells will agglutinate.

Agglutination-inhibition test

The fundamental agglutination reactions described above may be modified to form what is known as the agglutination-inhibition test. In this test, known X cells are mixed with known anti-X serum *after* the latter has been treated with the unknown antigen solution. If the expected agglutination reaction now fails to occur, it is inferred that soluble X antigen was present also in the unknown solution. The principle of this test is used in medico-legal work for identifying dried blood stains.

Action of incomplete antibodies

Incomplete antibodies are also known as blocking antibodies. In attaching themselves to cells, without causing agglutination, they prevent or block complete antibodies from doing so. This phenomenon has three important practical aspects.

(1) It explains many examples of prozoning. A prozone is a situation where neat antiserum, or even moderate dilutions of antiserum, will not cause agglutination while greater dilutions *will* cause it. The explanation for this remarkable effect is that the antiserum contains both complete and incomplete antibodies of the same specificity but of different titres, the incomplete antibody being of the lower titre. The incomplete antibody blocks the action of the complete antibody in the neat serum and in the low dilutions, but with progressive dilutions its activity is abolished, then the complete antibody goes into action.

(2) Occasionally a newborn baby, which is expected to be Rh positive, appears, on testing with complete anti-Rh serum, to be Rh negative. In fact, the baby is Rh positive, but it appears to be Rh negative because its Rh antigens have been blocked by the incomplete Rh antibodies derived from the mother. This fallacy would lead the doctor into a false sense of security if the direct Coombs test were not done.

(3) The above paradox (an Rh negative baby with Rh haemolytic disease) was first explained by Wiener, and on it he based a Blocking Test for incomplete Rh antibodies. In this test Rh positive cells are mixed with serum suspected of containing incomplete Rh antibodies. After a period of incubation they are washed and tested with complete Rh antiserum. If the expected agglutination fails to appear, it is inferred that incomplete Rh antibodies must have been present in the suspected antiserum. This was the first, and for some time the only, test for incomplete Rh antibodies. It is now replaced by the Coombs test.

LABORATORY ASPECTS

Coombs test—the antiglobulin test

There are two forms of this test, the direct and the indirect. The direct Coombs test is a test for incomplete antibodies attached to red cells. The cells are first washed several times and then mixed with Coombs reagent. Coombs reagent is anti-human globulin. If incomplete antibodies are attached to the cells, they, being human globulins, will react with the Coombs reagent and the cells will agglutinate. This test is used extensively in testing the red cells of newborn babies and in investigating cases of haemolytic anaemia.

In the indirect Coombs test, cells of known antigenic content (for example, Rh positive cells) are mixed with serum suspected of containing the corresponding incomplete antibodies. After a period of incubation, the cells are washed several times and then Coombs reagent is added as in the direct test. The cells are then examined for agglutination. If agglutination occurs it proves that the corresponding antibodies were present in the suspected serum. The indirect Coombs test is used mainly for checking the sera of pregnant women for incomplete Rh antibodies, and also in cross-matching tests prior to blood transfusion.

Haemolytic antibody reactions

Some antibodies, in the presence of complement, cause haemolysis of the red cells. Advantage is taken of this not only in detecting haemolytic antibodies, but also in detecting complement. In its simplest form, red cells, complement and antiserum are mixed together in a test tube and incubated at 37°C for a period. The test tube is then examined for haemolysis which, if present, indicates that an antigen-antibody reaction has taken place.

Complement fixation reactions

Sometimes an antigen-antibody reaction occurs which is completely invisible, but in the course of which all available complement is used up or fixed. This is called complement fixation. That complement is no longer available (in other words that an antigen-antibody reaction has occurred) is shown by adding red cells together with a haemolytic antibody. If haemolysis now takes place, then complement must have been available. Therefore there was no antigen-antibody reaction with the original ingredients. If, on the other hand, haemolysis does not take place, it means that there was no complement available; hence an antigen-antibody reaction must have taken place with the original ingredients.

The principle of complement fixation is used in a number of serological tests the best known of which is the Wasserman reaction for syphilis.

Coons fluorescent antibody test

In this test, which was introduced by Coons in 1941, a known antibody globulin is first conjugated with a fluorescent dye. When this conjugated antibody is placed in contact with its corresponding antigen, the resulting antigen-antibody complex shows up as a brilliant yellow-green fluorescence when observed under the microscope using ultraviolet light. The dyes commonly used for conjugation are fluorescein and rhodamine isothiocyanate. The latter is the more stable and gives the more brilliant fluorescence.

The Coons test has been used for the detection of antigens in bacteria, viruses, protozoa and fungi as well as human tissue antigens. There are two ways of applying the test in practice, the direct and indirect methods.

Direct method

In the direct method the antibody-dye conjugate is applied directly to the specimen under examination. Time is allowed for the antigen-antibody reaction to take place, and the excess antibody-dye conjugate is then removed by washing in buffered saline. The specimen is then mounted in glycerin and examined microscopically using ultraviolet light.

It will be apparent that in this method, separately conjugated antibody is required for each antigen sought. This difficulty is overcome in the indirect method.

Indirect method

Unconjugated antibody is applied to the specimen, time is allowed for the reaction to take place and then the excess antibody is washed off with buffered saline. Then anti-human globulin which has previously been conjugated with the dye, is added. At this point, the second antibody added, being an anti-globulin, will attach itself to the original antibody if it is present. The specimen is washed again, mounted, and examined. Thus, by using this method, only the anti-globulin need be conjugated.

The indirect Coons test should never be confused with the indirect Coombs test. The similarity is not only in the name.

Schultz-Dale reaction

In this experiment, smooth muscle is taken from an animal which is hypersensitive to, say, antigen X. The muscle is washed free of any circulating antibodies and is placed in a tissue bath with Ringer's solution. If antigen X is now added to the Ringer's solution in the bath, the muscle will contract. The extent of the contraction can be recorded by means of a kymograph lever on a moving drum. No antigen, other than antigen X, will cause the reaction.

A simpler modification of the test consists in excising a strip of smooth muscle from a normal animal. The uterus of a guinea-pig is often used. This muscle is made passively hypersensitive simply by soaking it in antiserum. The presence of this hypersensitivity can then be demonstrated in the tissue bath as described above.

6—Immunological responses

Having seen something of the nature of antigens in Chapter 1 and antibodies in Chapter 2, we now have to enquire into the effects of antigenic stimulation in Man. These effects are what are known as the immunological responses. There may be several different kinds of immunological response but at the present time three rather distinct and fairly well-defined responses are known.

Type 1 response (mainly protective)
Type 2 response (immediate hypersensitivity)
Type 3 response (delayed hypersensitivity)

MAINLY PROTECTIVE.

TYPE 1 RESPONSE—~~DELAYED HYPERSENSITIVITY~~

Type 1 response is the best known of the immunological responses. It is the one required when we vaccinate using foreign material (toxoids, attenuated viruses and so on but not BCG) for the purpose of protecting against infection. It is characterized by the production of circulating antibodies. For this reason it might be called the protective or prophylactic response. As the same response, however, occurs when there is no question of protection against disease (the iso-antibodies anti-A and anti-B) and indeed as the same response may actually *cause* disease (Rhesus disease) the name protective or prophylactic is not always appropriate—hence the non-committal term *Type 1 response* is used here. The term, however, does not imply that responses of this type are the first to occur after antigenic stimulation or that they are the most important.

Response to primary and secondary stimulation

The response to primary stimulation is delayed and when it occurs it is of low titre. This must not be confused with delayed hypersensi-

30

tivity. The antibody response to the second stimulation is immediate and of much higher titre. This must not be confused with immediate hypersensitivity. From these observations we conclude that the primary stimulation in some way prepares or educates the antibody-producing apparatus. By the time the second stimulation is given the education is complete—hence there is a quicker and more vigorous response. To begin with, the antibodies produced are of the Ig M type; later Ig G type antibodies are produced. The antibody titre achieved is not always the same or even similar. Some antigens are stronger than others and some persons react more vigorously to antigenic stimulation than others.

Natural immunity

In nature we are constantly exposed to various pathogenic organisms and sometimes we become infected with them, that is, we contract the disease. Sometimes the 'disease' is so mild that we hardly notice it—such infections are called sub-clinical. Whether the infection is clinical or sub-clinical, because the organisms possess antigens, we produce antibodies reactive against them. We are then immune to that disease for a variable length of time thereafter, sometimes for life. This is the basis of actively acquired natural immunity. Babies, on the other hand, who are incapable of producing antibodies, receive a ration of antibodies from the mother's blood before birth. This is known as passively acquired natural immunity and tides the baby over until such time as it can produce its own antibodies. The antibody-producing apparatus should be fully developed by six months of age.

TYPE 2 RESPONSE—IMMEDIATE HYPERSENSITIVITY

Type 2 response is the second great immunological response. Antigenic stimulation by one or more of a great variety of antigens (often called allergens in this connection) gives rise to a peculiar form of antibodies known as reagin or atopic antibodies. They are Ig E in type. These antibodies are peculiar in that they have a particular affinity for tissue cells to which they become attached and to which they may remain attached for years. This renders the tissue involved hypersensitive. They have a special affinity for skin tissue and are therefore often called *skin-sensitizing antibodies*. This title, while descriptive, is defective because the antibodies also form attachments to mucosae and smooth muscle especially the smooth muscle of the bronchi. They cannot be detected by agglutination, precipitation or complement fixation tests. Far from protecting against disease, these antibodies actually cause disease, indeed a high proportion of the average doctor's practice is made up of patients suffering from immediate hypersensitivity in one form or another.

Pathogenesis of immediate hypersensitivity reactions

After prolonged periods of stimulation by the antigens of grass pollen, animal dander, or house dust, the patient produces reagin antibodies which bind themselves to the tissues. Further exposure to the antigen causes an antigen-antibody reaction in, or on, the cells of the tissue involved. This reaction results in the liberation of highly active substances, mainly histamine, but also 5-hydroxytryptamine*, bradykinin and the so-called 'slow reacting factor' (SRF). After liberation, these substances exert their characteristic pharmacological effect. If the tissue involved is the smooth muscle of the bronchi, there will be bronchial constriction resulting in difficulty in breathing —for example, asthma and anaphylaxis. Should the mucous membrane of the nose and conjunctivae be involved there will be local hyperaemia and catarrh, a condition which is known clinically as hay fever. If the skin is involved, there may be a variety of rashes of which urticaria is the most significant.

Clinical importance of immediate hypersensitivity reactions

Immediate hypersensitivity responses are at the root of several disease entities in Man. The more important of these will be discussed in Chapter 8. By demonstrating the existence of immediate hypersensitivity to specific antigens and by appropriate desensitization much can be done to relieve these conditions.

Prausnitz-Kustner reaction

The Prausnitz-Kustner reaction gets its name from Prausnitz who performed the experiment with the cooperation of Kustner who was hypersensitive to fish. When some of Kustner's serum was injected into the skin of Prausnitz's arm, that area of the skin became hypersensitive to fish as was shown by the subsequent intradermal injection of fish extract into the site. In fact the antigen does not have to be injected; it may be taken by mouth when it will still cause the reaction. A varying period of up to 24 hours is necessary for the fixation of the antibodies to the skin but once fixed they remain there for four or five weeks.

From this reaction we see that immediate hypersensitivity can be

* Known as serotonin in the U.S.A.

transferred from one person to another by serum alone which shows that it is mediated by humeral factors (reagin antibody) and not by cells. Such a transfer is not possible with delayed hypersensitivity.

TYPE 3 RESPONSE—DELAYED HYPERSENSITIVITY

Delayed hypersensitivity is the third great immunological response which we must briefly consider at this point. In the early days of immunology Koch discovered that if he injected a healthy guinea-pig with tuberculin, nothing of note happened. If, however, he did the same thing to a guinea-pig which was already suffering from tuberculosis, something very much of note happened. There was both a general and a local reaction. The general reaction took the form of high temperature and malaise; the local reaction was an inflammation at the site of injection. These reactions did not occur immediately but about 24 hours after the injection was given. For this reason it was called delayed hypersensitivity. The time factor, however, is not the only, or indeed the most important point of difference between this response and the immediate hypersensitivity response. In the latter we saw that antibodies were involved—in this, there is no evidence of antibody involvement.

Proof of the immunological basis of delayed hypersensitivity

That the above phenomenon was caused by tuberculin might suggest that the reaction was toxic in origin and not immunological. The fact, however, that these reactions occur only after previous antigenic stimulation and the fact that they are specific both indicate that they are indeed immunological and not merely toxic reactions. That antibodies are not involved is shown by the fact that if serum from a positively reacting person is injected into the skin of a nega-tively reacting person, and if then, tuberculin is injected into the same site, there will still be no reaction. This contrasts with the situation in cases of immediate hypersensitivity.

Cell mediated response

If antibodies are not involved in this tuberculin reaction we are led to enquire into how it comes about. Microscopic examination of the skin lesion in these cases shows an infiltration with lympho-cytes and mononuclear cells together with a variable number of neutrophils. The most popular view concerning this cellular reaction is that the lymphocytes, which have 'memories' of previous

33

tuberculous infection, converge on the site of injection and accumulate there.

Clinical importance of delayed hypersensitivity reactions

The phenomenon of delayed hypersensitivity is utilized in the diagnosis of several diseases. It probably is profoundly involved in the pathogenesis of tuberculosis and other conditions, and it is the reaction responsible for the rejection of homografts. These aspects of the subject will be considered in Chapter 9.

Role of the thymus in immunological responses

That the thymus gland is concerned in immunological responses (especially Type 3 responses) is shown by the fact that removal of the thymus in newborn mice results in loss of ability to produce delayed hypersensitivity with consequent loss of ability to reject homografts. This is not the only effect of thymectomy in young mice but it is the most striking. Such mice may have their immunological potential restored by grafting thymus tissue from a normal mouse.

Further evidence of the important role of the thymus in immunological responses is obtained from observations on the Swiss type of congenital agammaglobulinaemia. In this condition there is aplasia of the thymus gland and associated with this there is a loss of all three types of immunological response. Such a condition is hardly compatible with life and indeed the patients usually die in early childhood. How exactly the thymus functions in regard to these immunological responses is still unknown.

That immune responses are far more complicated than was formerly thought is shown by the work of Miller and Globerson and Auerbach. Miller explored the role of the thymus in the immune response while Globerson and Auerbach discovered that antibody response to antigenic stimulation was produced *in vitro* only when cells of the thymus, bone marrow and (irradiated) spleen were present in the culture. This and other observations suggest that the immune response should be regarded as the resultant of the activity of at least three types of cells. In fact, three types of cells, macrophage, reactor cells and effector cells, each having a different function, are now involved in the immune response. The precise functional and cytogenetical relationship between these cell types is still unknown.

7—Diseases of the immunological apparatus

ANALYSIS

One of the ways of investigating the function of an organ is to extirpate the organ and observe how the animal fares without it. This method can hardly be applied to an organ such as the immunological apparatus, the cells of which are widely distributed throughout the body. Nature, however, has provided reasonable alternatives in certain diseases of the immunological apparatus. The study of these throws much light on what has been said up to now, particularly that on the role of antibodies and delayed hypersensitivity. These diseases will therefore be briefly considered, not in general, but only in so far as they are related to immunology.

Agammaglobulinaemia

Agammaglobulinaemia, or, as it is more correctly called, hypogammaglobulinaemia, is a condition in which the gammaglobulin content of the blood is greatly reduced. It may be so greatly reduced that it cannot be detected by ordinary paper electrophoresis, hence its original name, agammaglobulinaemia (*Figure 9*). More sensitive methods, however, show that there is nearly always some gammaglobulin present.

The normal gammaglobulin concentration ranges from about 600 to 1,500 mg per 100 ml of plasma. If it should fall below 200 mg per 100 ml, the case may be regarded as hypogammaglobulinaemia and treated as such.

The disease is suspected when a person, usually a young boy, suffers recurrent attacks of infection, often respiratory infection. It is confirmed by electrophoresis using the Grabar technique. Even with this technique, because a low Ig G may be masked by a high Ig M, it is advisable to use specific Ig G antiserum and not just anti-human globulin.

35

As might be anticipated, the disease is characterized by recurring bacterial infections and usually by defective blood groups. Defective blood groups are those in which the expected iso-antibodies are missing—for example a group A without the expected anti-B. But what is not anticipated is that patients with hypogammaglobulinaemia survive virus infections just as well as normal children. This observation rather reduces the significance of antibodies as far as virus infections are concerned.

Patients with hypogammaglobulinaemia seem to be able to tolerate homografts better than normal people, yet they are able to produce a delayed hypersensitivity reaction. This suggests that antibodies may play a small part in homograft rejection.

The treatment of the condition consists in the administration of gammaglobulin for as long as necessary, which usually means for life. More than ordinary care should be taken to avoid infection and all infections which are contracted should be promptly treated with antibiotics.

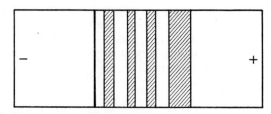

Figure 9 Serum electrophoresis in a case of hypo-gammaglobulinaemia. Note the absence of stain in the gamma globulin area. This appearance led to the condition being called 'agammaglobulinaemia'. In fact, some gamma globulin, too little to be detected by this test, is nearly always present. The condition is therefore more correctly called 'hypogammaglobulin-aemia'.

Thymus aplasia

In this rare condition there is aplasia of the thymus gland associated with generalized depletion of lymphoid tissue throughout the body. Even the lymphocytes of the blood are reduced.

There is, however, no defect in immunoglobulin production. The serum immunoglobulins attain normal levels and the patients can develop antibodies. Even though the patients can produce antibodies reactive against viruses, there is good evidence that their resistance to such infections is low. So once again the role of antibodies in virus infections is questioned. As might be expected, patients with this disease tolerate homografts and appear to be unable to develop delayed hypersensitivity. Thus the role of delayed hypersensitivity in homograft rejection is once again underlined.

Swiss type of agammaglobulinaemia

The Swiss type of agammaglobulinaemia may be regarded as a combination of the two conditions already discussed. There is thus a marked deficiency of gamma globulin, all the immunoglobulins being involved, together with depletion of lymphoid tissue throughout the body.

Patients with this condition are, as might be expected, prone to bacterial and virus disease. The disease, in these circumstances, is hardly compatible with life. All reported cases died before the age of two years.

Functional deficiency of immunoglobulin

In these cases the concentration of immunoglobulins in the serum is within normal limits yet the patients behave as though they were cases of hypogammaglobulinaemia. Thus, one patient was reported to have had 600 chest infections, but to have improved on treatment with gamma globulin. This observation would suggest that although the immunoglobulins are present in normal amounts, they are functionally deficient. These cases probably represent a defect in immunoglobulin synthesis which involves that part of the molecule which normally combines with the antigen.

Such cases cannot be recognized by electrophoresis because, as already mentioned, the immunoglobulin level in the serum is normal. When a patient, suspected of having hypogammaglobulinaemia, is found to have normal serum levels of immunoglobulin, the true condition can be brought to light by injecting an antigen and observing whether or not the corresponding antibody appears.

Myelomatosis

In this condition there is a malignant proliferation of plasma cells which is associated with a high protein content in the blood serum. This high protein content is often first manifested by excessive rouleaux formation as seen in a blood film. Any of the immunoglobulins may, in theory, be involved in the increase but by far the commonest is Ig G. The increase in Ig G is associated with a decrease in the other immunoglobulins. This is in harmony with the belief that the malignant proliferation stems from a single, or single group of plasma cells, and it explains why the condition is often referred to as a monoclonal gammopathy.

Ordinary paper electrophoresis shows a dense narrow band in the gamma or beta globulin area of the strip (*Figure 10*). Further investigation by the immunoelectrophoresis technique of Grabar or the double diffusion technique of Ouchterlony, will show which immunoglobulin is involved.

An attempt has been made to correlate the immunoglobulin type with the clinical picture—thus the Ig G type is said to be associated with immune paresis, the Ig A type with hypercalcaemia and renal failure, and the Ig M type with the viscosity syndrome.

Waldenstrom's macroglobulinaemia

In this disease, which is similar to myelomatosis, there is a proliferation of lymphocytes rather than plasma cells. Although Waldenstrom suggested the name 'incipient myelomatosis' for the condition, it has been regarded as a lymphosarcoma because of the lymphocytic proliferation.

It is characterized clinically by bleeding from the nose and gums. In about 50 per cent of cases there is enlargement of the lymphatic glands, the liver and the spleen. Macroglobulin is found in the serum and this leads to increased viscosity of the blood and a strong tendency to form rouleaux. This latter is often noticed on the blood film and it immediately suggests that a full examination of the serum proteins should be undertaken. In this way the disease is brought to light.

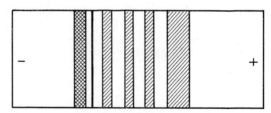

Figure 10 Serum electrophoresis in a case of myelomatosis. Note the dense and narrow stain in the gamma globulin area. This indicates not only a greater concentration of gamma globulin but also gamma globulin of a more homogeneous kind.

As in myelomatosis and lupus erythematosus, the Sia test is often positive. Macroglobulin forms up to 50 per cent of the total serum proteins but, unlike cases of myelomatosis there is no particular susceptibility to infection.

8—Immediate hypersensitivity

That certain people react in an untoward manner to otherwise harmless substances is a fact that has been known for well over 100 years. These untoward reactions usually take the form of bronchial asthma, hay fever, urticaria, eczema or, more uncommonly, anaphylaxis. Very often two or more of these reactions occur together in an individual case.

The number of substances which can give rise to such reactions are legion: no good purpose would be served by attempting to list them all, but the following should be remembered. Grass pollen, especially Timothy and Ragwort, is particularly important. Animal dander, fish, fruit, house dust, penicillin, aspirin and many other drugs have been incriminated. So commonly do these immediate hypersensitivity reactions occur after exposure to pollen that, in certain cities of the world, a pollen count in the atmosphere is done, and the results are broadcast as a subject of news.

PSYCHOLOGICAL COMPLICATIONS

Psychological reactions may, and often do, manifest themselves in the same way as allergic reactions. Thus, for example, a variety of psychological factors may bring about asthma and urticaria. Repressed resentment, in particular, may be just as potent a cause of asthma as pollen. These complications lead to confusion, especially in the mind of the laity. There is, of course, no reason why a person who is hypersensitive to pollen should not also have resentments which he suppresses, but it is important to separate the two in theory even if it proves to be impossible to do so in practice. Stress may cause asthma, but it does not cause allergy. Allergy is caused by antigens.

In trying to decide whether a given reaction is allergic or psychological in origin, some help may be obtained from a differential white cell count. Allergy is often associated with eosinophilia.

The problem deepens

It has been said above that it is important, in theory at least, to separate the two factors, psychological and allergic, which may give rise to, for example, asthma. This is because much time and money may be wasted doing skin tests, diet elimination tests, and even carrying out desensitization programmes on persons who are not allergic but psychological cases. It has also been suggested that it may not be possible to separate the two in practice. Cases have been reported in which a patient, allergic to geraniums, had asthmatic attacks on being presented with artificial geraniums. Another patient, who was allergic to horse dander, had asthmatic attacks whenever he saw a photograph of a horse. Such cases are probably examples of conditioning along Pavlovian lines.

EXAMPLES OF IMMEDIATE HYPERSENSITIVITY

Asthma

Asthma is characterized by recurrent attacks of wheezing often, and typically, with difficulty in breathing. Attacks vary greatly from mild to severe. Between attacks the patient may appear quite normal but eventually secondary changes, such as chronic bronchitis and emphysema, set in. Emphysema leads to increased pulmonary blood pressure and finally to heart failure. The presence of an eosinophilia will suggest an allergic rather than a psychological cause for the asthma.

For moderate to severe attacks, adrenaline is the drug of choice in the majority of cases. Ephedrine, because it has the advantage that it can be taken by mouth, may be substituted in selected cases. Prednisone is of great value in status asthmaticus and it may also be used to prevent attacks in chronic asthmatics.

In 1967, Altounyan showed that inhalation of disodium cromoglycate inhibited allergic asthma. This observation has been confirmed many times since. Cromoglycate is believed to act by inhibiting the release of histamine and SRS from tissue cells.

From the purely immunological point of view, the most exciting discovery was that of Ishizaka who showed that the reagin antibody was of the Ig E type. This discovery led to promising attempts at blocking sensitization of the cells by means of non-allergen-specific

Ig E. Such cells would therefore be protected from the effects of allergen-specific Ig E.

Urticaria

Urticaria may result from the ingestion, inhalation or parental administration of the offending antigen. In hospital practice it is often seen after a blood transfusion. The history of the attack often indicates the source of the antigen and therefore the action which should be taken to prevent such attacks in the future. In some cases it is necessary to resort to skin testing but this should only be done when psychological factors can be reasonably excluded.

The acute attack usually yields to treatment with antihistamine but occasionally steroid hormones may be required.

Hay fever

Hay fever is not serious, but it is an irritating condition and it is exceedingly common. It usually takes the form of sneezing, running from the eyes and nose, and itching of the eyes. Sometimes mild asthma occurs also.

The treatment is not satisfactory and many patients, including patients who are themselves doctors, just learn to live with their malady. In more irritating cases, skin testing, followed by desensitization may be tried.

Penicillin hypersensitivity

The number of people who are hypersensitive to penicillin must run into millions. In the United States alone, it is reported that there are 300 deaths from this cause each year. This says little of the non-fatal illness which can be attributed to it.

Modes of acquiring the hypersensitivity

The high frequency of penicillin hypersensitivity is due to the widespread use of penicillin not only by injection but also in the form of ointments, creams and lozenges. Other, less obvious, ways include the following.

(1) Drinking milk which contains penicillin.
(2) The use of vaccines which contain penicillin.
(3) The use of syringes contaminated with penicillin.
(4) Handling or inhaling penicillin.

Clinical manifestations of penicillin hypersensitivity

When taken by mouth, the hypersensitivity may manifest itself by typical allergic reactions on the lips or mucous membranes of the mouth and pharynx. Oedema of the larynx is a special danger. When the drug is absorbed it may cause an irritating generalized urticaria and sometimes angioneurotic oedema. When the penicillin is given by injection there may be breathlessness, collapse and death.

Prevention of penicillin reactions

Any person who gives a history of penicillin hypersensitivity must not receive penicillin. In the majority of cases a suitable alternative antibiotic can be found. Penicillin, because of its potency in causing hypersensitivity, should always be used with circumspection and not for trivial infections. Adrenaline, which is the main treatment for the serious cases, should always be readily available whenever penicillin is being administered.

Treatment of penicillin hypersensitivity reactions

The treatment follows the same lines as for any other allergic reaction. Adrenaline is the main drug in serious cases. If there is collapse it should be given intramuscularly at the rate of a minim a minute. Steroid hormones and antihistaminics may be given later if required.

Penicillinase in the treatment of penicillin reactions

Penicillinase is among the most potent enzymes known. By catalytic hydrolysis it converts penicillin into penicilloic acid which is non-antigenic. Its value in the treatment of penicillin reactions has been confirmed many times and the results are often quite dramatic. It may be used alone but it is often used in conjunction with steroid hormones.

SKIN TESTING IN IMMEDIATE HYPERSENSITIVITY

If you approach skin testing with the idea that you will always get crisp unequivocal results, you are bound to be disappointed. In the vast majority of cases there will be no such result. Nevertheless, in some cases the results are most revealing and this is the justification for the use of skin testing in all moderate or severe cases of immediate hypersensitivity.

Dangers of skin testing

Skin testing is always a tedious and rather painful procedure and, what is far more important, unless it is done with circumspection it may cause alarming anaphylactic reactions which are sometimes fatal. Because of this, a routine of testing which minimizes discomfort and lessens the risk of severe reactions should be followed. The entire routine is best learnt in a department or clinic which specializes in the work.

Routine procedure

Different centres have slightly different routine procedures. The following is suggested as fairly typical.

(1) A detailed history of the hypersensitivity reaction should be taken. This is essential. Such a history will sometimes bring to light an allergen against which the patient reacts violently. This allergen must not be used in the tests.

(2) Scratch tests should always be done before intradermal tests. Scratch tests are not as sensitive as intradermal tests, but they are also not as dangerous. Allergens which give strong reactions with the scratch test should not be used for the intradermal test.

(3) The flexor surface of the forearm is the most convenient site for intradermal testing. A different needle and syringe should be used for each allergen. It is important to use a control consisting of the extracting solution without the allergen. This will reveal reactions to chemicals in the solution and also the odd case of dermographia.

(4) Adrenaline, antihistamine and aminophylline should be immediately available lest, despite the above precautions, the patient still has a severe reaction. If, as so often happens, the patient is already taking antihistamine, it should be discontinued a day or preferably two days before skin testing.

Interpretation of the results

If care is taken with the whole procedure, there should be a good correlation between the results of the skin tests and the clinical history. Sometimes, however, there is no such correlation. The various combinations found are listed below together with possible explanations for discrepancies and the action to be taken.

(1) *Positive clinical history with positive skin tests*

A definite diagnosis can be made and desensitization begun.

(2) *Positive clinical history with negative skin tests*

Negative skin reactions are sometimes found in combination with a highly suggestive clinical history. This may be due to the use of inactive allergens. Allergens obtained from a reliable source only should be used. This combination is found mainly in relation to pollens when the target tissue is the mucous membrane of the nose or bronchi. For these cases it may be necessary to resort to mucosal testing. If the clinical history is highly suggestive, desensitization may be tried despite the negative skin tests.

(3) Negative clinical history with positive skin tests

This combination may be due to what is called latent sensitization. Such cases often give a positive clinical history in the future. It may also be due to a cross-reacting allergen. In either event, do not attempt desensitization, advise against contact with the allergen suggested by the skin test and any possible cross-reacting allergens. Keep the patient under observation.

Desensitization in immediate hypersensitivity

Desensitization (or hyposensitization) means the abolition (or lessening) of the antigen-antibody reaction by immunological means. This definition excludes such relief as may be obtained from the use of adrenaline, steroid hormones, antihistaminics and so on. Desensitization consists in the administration of graded doses of the offending antigen. The material is best given by subcutaneous injection. It has been used successfully in the treatment of immediate hypersensitivity due to a wide range of antigens of both animal and vegetable origin. It cannot, of course, be used if the antigen also happens to be a toxin.

For pollen, and other seasonal hypersensitivities, the injections are most effective if they are given prior to the season in which the antigen appears. In practice, this means that treatment should be commenced about three months before the pollen season. The injections are usually continued until the patient's skin test for the antigen becomes negative. The great disadvantage of this procedure is that it is tedious for both doctor and patient and indeed many patients default in their treatment.

More recently, instead of an aqueous extract of the antigen, an alum-precipitated pyridine extract has been used. As this preparation is more slowly absorbed, bigger doses may be given and at longer intervals with the result that the total number of injections is greatly reduced. Patients, especially children, find this much more acceptable. Clinical trials show these extracts to be at least as effective and possibly even more effective than the older aqueous extracts. The alum-precipitated pyridine extracts are available in England under the name 'Allpyral'. The mixed grass extract contains cocksfoot, meadow fescue, perennial rye, Timothy and Yorkshire fog.

The precise mechanism of desensitization is unknown. It has been suggested that injections of the offending antigen stimulate the production not of reagin, but of ordinary antibodies and that these neutralize or block the antigen before it can react with the reagin antibody which is fixed to the tissues.

9—Delayed hypersensitivity

ANALYSIS OF DELAYED HYPERSENSITIVITY

Delayed hypersensitivity, or, as it is sometimes called, cellular hypersensitivity, is the third great immunological response which we have to consider. It is also the most difficult to understand.

From its common name we get the idea that a time lag or delay distinguishes this form of hypersensitivity. That is correct. In immediate hypersensitivity the response occurs within a few minutes of contact with the antigen, but in this form of hypersensitivity there is a delay of several hours before the response becomes apparent. The time factor is by no means the only, nor indeed is it the most important, difference between immediate and delayed hypersensitivity —it is, however, the most obvious.

Contrast between immediate and delayed hypersensitivity

Far more significant than the time factor is the fact that while immediate hypersensitivity can be transmitted from one person to another by transferring the serum, delayed hypersensitivity cannot be transmitted in this way but only by the transfer of lymphoid cells. This shows that a distinctly different mechanism is at work in delayed hypersensitivity. While immediate hypersensitivity is caused by antibodies (reagin) delayed hypersensitivity is caused by cells or possibly by cell-bound antibodies. Table 3 shows further distinguishing features between these two forms of hypersensitivity.

Tuberculin reaction

Tuberculosis has become the prototype of delayed hypersensitivity and the tuberculin reaction has become the prototype of its skin manifestation. A person who has, or who has had tuberculosis or a person who has been vaccinated with BCG, is in a state of delayed hypersensitivity in regard to tuberculoprotein. This is manifested in the skin by means of the tuberculin test.

47

TABLE 3

	Immediate hypersensitivity	Delayed hypersensitivity
Time lapse	a few minutes	several hours
Transferred by serum	Yes	No
Transferred by cells	No	Yes
Useful to the body	No	Yes (?)
Inhibited by antihistamine	Yes	No

If a small amount of tuberculoprotein is injected intradermally in a person who is in a state of delayed hypersensitivity, a local area of redness and induration appears at the site of injection some 12 to 36 hours later. This lasts for a few days, then it gradually subsides. If excess tuberculoprotein is injected there may be, in addition, ulceration at the site. No such reaction takes place in the non-hypersensitive person.

Microscopic appearance of the lesion

Descriptions of the microscopic appearance of the tuberculin reaction vary greatly. This is undoubtedly because the lesion is not static but constantly changing. Hence the appearance at one time may be quite different from that a few hours later. Initially there is a moderate inflammatory reaction with the exudation of neutrophils. A few hours later the neutrophils have migrated and are replaced by mononuclear cells (lymphocytes and monocytes) which first appear in the perivascular tissue. Later still there is a further exudation of neutrophils. In the meantime, local oedema occurs and in severe cases necrosis, resulting in ulceration, takes place. In short, the picture is that of acute inflammation with strong shades of chronic inflammation.

Is delayed hypersensitivity protective in nature?

This question has been debated for many years. At first sight it seems that delayed hypersensitivity is a distinct hazard, leading on reinfection, to a local area of inflammation with necrosis, ulceration, and loss of tissue, none of which would occur in the non-hypersensitive person. On the other hand, the hypersensitivity, leading as it does to the prompt mobilization of cells (including phagocytes) and their localization in the reinfected area, helps to rid the body of the offending antigen. Payling Wright says, 'In brief, the loss of a small mass of necrosed tissue at the point of reinfection . . . seems a small price to pay for localizing and perhaps eliminating a potentially dangerous invader.'

Immunity in tuberculosis

This leads on to a consideration of immunity in tuberculosis, a problem which, even after many years of study, is still unsolved. If an animal is vaccinated with BCG it produces antibodies, it enters a state of delayed hypersensitivity, and it develops a relative, but not absolute, immunity to tuberculosis. The first thought that naturally comes to mind is that the antibodies cause both the hypersensitivity and the immunity. Experiments, however, show that it is not possible to transmit either the hypersensitivity or the immunity from one individual to another by transferring the serum. The antibodies, therefore, do not seem to be concerned with either the hypersensitivity or the immunity. Furthermore, it is possible, by means of repeated injections of tuberculoprotein, to remove the hypersensitivity without removing the immunity. We therefore may conclude that the hypersensitivity is not part and parcel, but distinct from, the immunity. All this suggests that the immunity is to be sought in the cells. Undoubtedly the phagocytes are there, undoubtedly they phagocytose the invaders, yet they often seem to do more harm than good.

Delayed hypersensitivity in the pathogenesis of tuberculosis

The tubercle bacillus is a remarkably bland organism. It is slow to grow, it does not move and it does not produce toxins. How then can it be among the most deadly of Man's enemies? Before considering this question two pertinent observations will be made. Penicillin is a remarkably bland and non-toxic substance, yet it is the most lethal drug in the doctor's bag. Horse serum is a bland substance but we shall see something of the harm it can cause in anaphylaxis, serum sickness and the Arthus phenomenon. Could something similar apply to the tubercle bacillus? A study of the reactions of the tissues to this organism from early tubercle formation, through caseation and ulceration, to acute disseminated tuberculosis is not incompatible with this suggestion. In other words, tuberculosis may be essentially an allergic disease brought about by hypersensitivity to the tubercle bacillus.

Delayed hypersensitivity in other conditions

Apart from infections, delayed hypersensitivity may occur as a result of contact with a number of chemical substances (including drugs) and plants. In these cases the hypersensitivity is manifested by what is commonly called *contact dermatitis*. This begins as a papular lesion which becomes vesicular. Then it weeps, crusts form and finally there may be hyperkeratosis. A similar reaction is seen in persons undergoing secondary vaccination for smallpox. This, though an example of delayed hypersensitivity, is confusingly called the immediate reaction.

Advantage is taken of the presence of delayed hypersensitivity in the diagnosis of several chronic infectious diseases. This will be considered in Chapter 15.

Homograft rejection

A homograft is a graft taken from one individual and grafted to another individual of the same species. The great problem with homografting is that the grafted tissue or organ is nearly always destroyed and rejected. That this phenomenon is immunological in nature is not doubted. Some doubt, however, exists as to which particular immunological response is involved.

Is homograft rejection due to Type 1 response?

The homograft contains many proteins which are foreign to the recipient. In addition to this, antibodies of various kinds have been detected in the serum of recipients following homografting. These antibodies, however, are not invariably found and the consensus of opinion is that they play little, if any, part in the rejection process. That persons with hypogammaglobulinaemia are slow to reject homografts is a tantalizing fact.

Is homograft rejection due to immediate hypersensitivity?

There is nothing to suggest that homograft rejection is due to immediate hypersensitivity. The phenomenon is not transferable by serum.

Is homograft rejection due to delayed hypersensitivity?

Microscopic examination of the rejected tissue shows infiltration, sometimes intense infiltration, with mononuclear cells such as are seen in cases of indubitably delayed hypersensitivity reactions. Furthermore, the ability to reject homografts in an accelerated form, has been transmitted from one individual to another by transferring certain lymphoid cells. For these reasons it is believed that delayed hypersensitivity is the main, if not the only, factor in homograft rejection.

Delayed hypersensitivity and malignant growth

Even in the early days of immunology it was believed that there was a strong connection between immune processes and malignant growth. This belief was based largely on the work of Ehrlich, Bashford and Wade. Thus, writing in 1908, Wade said, 'The tumour is borne away on a lymphocytic tide.' He was speaking of a transplanted tumour, but he seems to be describing delayed hypersensitivity. Other evidence of an association between delayed hypersensitivity and malignant growth may be summarized as follows.

(1) There is a greater frequency of malignant growth in patients with a negative Mantoux reaction than in those with a positive Mantoux reaction. Hughes and Mackay report that only about 50 per cent of their cancer patients gave positive results on tuberculin testing while some 90 per cent of control patients reacted positively.

(2) There is a delay in the rejection of homografts of malignant tissue in patients who already have malignant tumours. This observation suggests an inhibition of delayed hypersensitivity in patients with malignant growths.

(3) The success of transplanting a homograft depends largely on the inability of the recipient to develop delayed hypersensitivity. This applies to malignant as well as to normal tissue.

(4) The prognosis of patients with malignancy seems to depend, among other things, on their ability or inability to develop delayed hypersensitivity. Those who cannot do so have a worse prognosis than those who can.

(5) The microscopic appearance of many malignant lesions has features similar to those of delayed hypersensitivity; indeed a lymphocytic reaction around the malignant growth has been related favourably to prognosis.

(6) The artificial suppression of delayed hypersensitivity has been associated with an increased incidence of malignant growth.

10—Allergy

A CHAPTER OF CONFUSION

Immunity, hyperimmunity, sensitivity, hypersensitivity, prophylaxis, anaphylaxis, anaphylactoid—these are some of the terms used in connection with the subject-matter of this book. They have, however, become so blunted by misuse throughout the years that they convey neither their original meaning nor any generally accepted meaning. In short, they have become vague. This has led to further confusion in a subject already confused by nature.

Realizing the difficulty in the early days of immunology, von Pirquet coined the term 'allergy' to cover all these forms of changed reactivity that we have been discussing up until now. In the English translation by Carl Prausnitz, he says 'For this general concept of *changed* reactivity I propose the term "allergy".' Nothing could be more clear.

De-confusion

The term 'allergic' therefore is correctly applied to an individual who has been protected against disease and also to an individual who, as a result of antigenic stimulation, reacts in an untoward way to further stimulation by that antigen subsequently. The child who has been vaccinated against smallpox is thus allergic to the smallpox virus, just as the person who develops hay fever on exposure to pollen is allergic to pollen. The term 'immune' should be used to denote protection against disease, while the term 'hypersensitivity' should be used to denote such untoward reactions as hay fever, asthma, anaphylaxis, and so on, which follow repeated exposure to an antigen. The situation is graphically represented as follows.

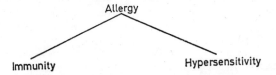

The term 'sensitive' seems to be used synonymously with 'hypersensitive' and is therefore redundent. Similarly, the term 'prophylaxis' is used synonymously with 'immunity' so it, too, is redundant. Anaphylactoid may be applied to reactions similar to anaphylaxis which do not have an allergic basis.

Combined immunity and hypersensitivity

All this does not mean that the two conditions, immunity and hypersensitivity, are mutually exclusive. Richet's dogs, as we shall see, were both immune and hypersensitive to the toxin of actinaria. But the rabbits of Arthus were purely hypersensitive as the question of protection against disease is irrelevant.

There is a further difficulty at this point. To the particular kind of hypersensitivity which he induced in his dogs, Richet applied the term 'anaphylaxis'. By this he meant to imply a concept opposite in meaning to immunity, to use his own words 'L'anaphylaxie signifie le contraire de la protection'. This led to the extraordinary paradox of his dogs being immune and not immune at the same time. By viewing the situation in the terms described above (that is, by regarding anaphylaxis as a form of hypersensitivity) the paradox is resolved.

Other difficulties

Now other difficulties arise. von Pirquet must have known about the ABO blood groups but he certainly could not have known about the rhesus groups. Is a group A person allergic to group B blood? As the group A person has developed anti-B since his birth (in other words as his reactivity has changed) I think von Pirquet would say that he was allergic. Is a rhesus negative woman who has rhesus antibodies in her serum, allergic to rhesus positive blood? Again, I think von Pirquet would say that she was, but he would have to add that the allergy manifests itself, not in her,* but in her baby.

Is all this a quibble?

It is often said that words are not important provided you know

* Unless she received a transfusion of rhesus positive blood.

what you mean and what you are talking about. This sounds trite, but it is worse than that—it is incorrect. Words are the things we think with, hence if our words are wrong or muddled then our thinking is likely to be wrong and muddled too.

Do I practise what I preach?

No. The very title of this book is a transgression of the principles advocated in the above paragraphs. I should have called it, were I a man of principle, *A Primer of Allergy*. Had I done so, however, I would have conveyed the wrong idea of its contents to the vast majority of the medical profession who see in allergy a sort of twilight, almost mystical science, which concerns itself with such things as pollen, feathers, skin scratches and asthma. The law of English is that usage, even incorrect usage, determines meaning. I choose to remain within the law, but I urge my readers to break it.

A bird's eye view of Allergy and its Relatives

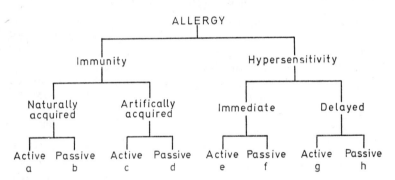

Examples

(*a*) Clinical and sub-clinical infections such as measles, rubella, poliomyelitis.

(*b*) Immunity acquired passively *in utero* from the mother against such infections as measles, rubella, poliomyelitis and so on.

(*c*) Immunity artificially produced by various vaccines, smallpox, diphtheria, whooping cough and so on.

(*d*) Passive immunity given by means of antisera from other animals and used mainly for diphtheria cases and contacts and those with wounds which might result in tetanus.

(*e*) Hay fever, urticaria, allergic asthma, anaphylaxis, serum sickness.

(*f*) The Prausnitz-Kustner reaction.
(*g*) The hypersensitivity following infection with tubercle bacilli and so on.
(*h*) An experimental procedure, following the transfer of lymphoid cells.

No biological classification is ever completely satisfactory; hence, while they may be useful to begin with, they should never be slavishly followed. There are three well-known allergic reactions which, though always cited as examples of immediate hypersensitivity, do not fall comfortably into this or any other category. These three are—the Arthus phenomenon, Richet's phenomenon (anaphylaxis), and serum sickness. From the classical descriptions, these do not appear to be immediate but indeed very delayed reactions, so confusion once again arises. For this, and other reasons, these reactions are best considered separately and not included, to begin with at any rate, with the established forms of hypersensitivity such as that caused by pollen.

Arthus phenomenon

Arthus discovered that repeated subcutaneous injections of horse serum into a rabbit eventually led to an area of intense inflammation with, in some cases, necrosis and ulceration. As the whole process may take weeks to develop, it is, understandably, difficult to see why it is called an immediate reaction. An appreciation of the pathogenesis of the condition, however, largely resolves this difficulty. At the same time, however, it shows other reasons why this type of reaction is better divorced from the usual (for example, pollen) types of immediate hypersensitivity.

To begin with, Arthus was dealing with a non-allergic animal and the first few injections merely served to create the allergic state. This took the form of the animal developing, not reagin type antibodies as, for example, with pollen, but ordinary circulating precipitating antibodies. Now, when the final injection is given, a remarkable series of events takes place. The antigen is deposited in the subcutaneous tissue and is thus separated from the circulating antibody by the small blood vessel walls. In their attempt to reach one another, antigen and antibody create havoc. The endothelial lining of the blood vessels swells, platelets and neutrophils clump together, stasis of the blood occurs, then thrombosis and necrosis, small vessels rupture, there is haemorrhage and finally ulceration.

Studies by immunofluorescence show that an antigen-antibody reaction has taken place in the actual walls of the vessels.

We see, therefore, that apart from the question of time, this reaction differs from pollen hypersensitivity in that it is mediated by precipitating antibodies and also in that the lesion is far more cellular and far more destructive.

Anaphylaxis (Richet's phenomenon)

Richet discovered that on giving a certain dose of a toxic extract of actinaria to dogs, nothing of note happened. But, on giving the same dose some days later, some of his dogs died. He was not misled into thinking that death was due to the cumulative effect of the toxin. He recognized that the animals which had died had changed their reactivity to the extract and for this change he coined the word *anaphylaxis*. Theobald Smith made the same discovery independently but in this case the results were more convincing because Smith was working, not with a toxic substance, but with normal horse serum.

The precise mechanism of anaphylaxis is still not clear. The following, however, is a working account. Injections of foreign protein lead to the formation of antibodies. Some of these antibodies become attached to tissue cells, others circulate in the blood stream. On further injection, the protein is carried in the blood stream to the organs where the antibodies are attached. When antigen meets antibody, a reaction takes place which results in the liberation of pharmacologically active substances the most important of which is histamine. The liberated histamine then brings about the characteristic changes which we call anaphylaxis. Anaphylaxis differs from one animal species to another but it is always similar to acute histamine poisoning in a given animal.

It has also been shown that intravenous injection of antigen-antibody complexes may result in anaphylaxis. This observation suggests an alternative pathogenetic mechanism, for it seems possible that the circulating antibodies formed as a result of the first injection may combine with the antigen given in the second injection, and that the antigen-antibody complex so formed brings about the anaphylactic reaction.

Serum sickness

von Pirquet and Schick discovered that as a result of administering large doses of anti-diphtheria serum (obtained from horses) to patients, the patients sometimes developed a peculiar sickness after a period of about a week. This manifested itself by pyrexia, urticaria, lymph glandular swellings and pains in the joints. They called it serum sickness.

A consideration of the pathogenesis of the condition will reveal why a reaction which occurs after a delay of a week, is regarded as an example of immediate hypersensitivity. The patient, to begin with, is not allergic. The injection of the horse serum first produces reagin type antibodies and these become attached to various tissues, skin, joints and so on. The patient is now allergic. Because the initial dose of antigen was so large, some antigen is still present after the allergic state is established, and this antigen reacts with the reagin antibody which is attached to the tissues. Immediately after contact of antigen with attached antibody, histamine is released and symptoms follow. Later, precipitating antibodies appear. These combine with the remaining antigen and the symptoms begin to disappear.

How does the practitioner stand in regard to these phenomena?

In the days when von Pirquet and Schick described serum sickness (1900) the use of antisera in the treatment of diphtheria was in its infancy. Large doses of the antiserum had to be given to obtain the desired result. Today, far more potent and refined antisera are available, large doses are not necessary and serum sickness is an almost negligible problem. Nevertheless, foreign proteins or protein fractions are present in the antiserum and with them, the possibility of unfavourable immunological reactions. A case can therefore be made for the production of antisera (against diphtheria and tetanus) in human beings. This, however, raises the problem of homologous serum jaundice—a disease which is far worse than serum sickness. But with the solution of this problem, the suggestion that antisera be obtained from human sources becomes more feasible.

At one time anaphylaxis was merely a laboratory phenomenon and though it was, and still is, a source of irritation for those trying to produce antiserum in animals, it was not a clinical problem of importance. Those days have passed. With the ever-increasing number of drugs available, notably penicillin, we can confidently, if reluctantly, look forward to an increasing incidence of anaphylaxis. Every practitioner should therefore always have immediately available those drugs required for the treatment of anaphylaxis.

Although mild cases of the Arthus phenomenon may occur from time to time in medical practice, they present no particular problem and indeed may often remain unrecognized. Generally speaking, the Arthus phenomenon may be regarded in the same way as anaphylaxis was in the past, a laboratory affair. In the production of anti-lymphocyte serum in horses, for example, most workers used the subcutaneous route for the injections. This has led to severe Arthus phenomena sometimes with the death of the horses. Intravenous injection, on the other hand, has produced anaphylaxis.

Farmer's lung as an Arthus phenomenon

Farmer's lung is a pneumonia-like condition which follows repeated exposure to mouldy vegetable matter, especially mouldy hay. Hay becomes mouldy as a result of being stored while still damp. It is thus a common occurrence during wet summers and this corresponds with the incidence of Farmer's lung. Mouldy hay is virtually a culture of thermophilic actinomycetes, notably Micropolyspora faeni.

Pathogenesis of Farmer's lung

Repeated inhalation of the mould organisms leads to the development of precipitating antibodies reactive against a watery extract of mouldy hay. This reasonably suggested that the pathological changes which follow in the lungs are, in fact, due to an Arthus phenomenon. A similar pathogenetic mechanism is probably responsible for bagassosis (mouldy sugar cane) and other conditions where organic matter is repeatedly inhaled.

11—Immunohaematology

For an understanding of the chapters which follow, a certain knowledge of blood groups and other aspects of immunohaematology is required. In the past 20 years, knowledge of blood groups has accumulated to such a vast extent that it has far out-stripped the requirements of clinical medicine. Thus, at the present time, some 14 different blood group systems are known and yet only two of these, the ABO and the Rhesus systems, have regular application in medical practice, and not all that is known about these two systems is really relevant. In the following chapters, therefore, I have tried to sort the wheat from the chaff and thus to present what seems to me to be the most important aspects of the subject. The main criterion of importance has been relevance to medical practice.

ABO BLOOD GROUP SYSTEM

Several features of this blood group system have already been mentioned in illustration of certain points about antigens and antibodies. Here, it is necessary to pursue the subject in greater detail.

The ABO blood groups are determined by the use of the two naturally occurring iso-antibodies, anti-A and anti-B, which are found in group B and group A blood respectively. In this test, the unknown cells are added to the two known antisera, incubated and then examined for agglutination. This is called the major grouping. In theory, the use of two antisera can always give rise to four possible

Anti-A	Anti-B		
+	−	=	Group A
−	+	=	Group B
+	+	=	Group AB
−	−	=	Group O

results and this theoretical possibility is realized in the present situation.

In practice, not only are the cells tested for their antigens—the serum is also tested for its antibody content. This is known as the minor grouping and is done by the use of group A and group B cells.

A cells	B cells		
−	+	=	Group A
+	−	=	Group B
−	−	=	Group AB
+	+	=	Group O

Landsteiner's rule says that whenever an antigen is absent from the cell, the corresponding antibody is present in the serum. This rule is applicable only to the ABO system and with few exceptions it is valid. The minor grouping, therefore, is an almost perfect check of the major grouping.

Third antibody—anti-C

The above reactions are implied in the simple table given on page 8. Though sufficient for most practical purposes they nevertheless leave some phenomena unexplained. Thus, when a group O serum is absorbed with group A cells, it loses not only its anti-A activity but also some of its anti-B activity. Similarly, when it is absorbed with B cells, it loses not only its anti-B but also some of its anti-A. Furthermore, if a group O person is injected with A cells (or A substance) his anti-B titre rises as well as his anti-A. If he is injected with B cells, his anti-A titre rises as well as his anti-B.

As these findings cannot be explained in terms of this table, Wiener extended the concept as shown in Table 4.

TABLE 4

Blood group	Antigens present	Antibodies present
A	A and C	Anti-B
B	B and C	Anti-A
AB	A, B and C	—
O	Nil	Anti-A, Anti-B and Anti-C

There is a third antibody, anti-C, in group O serum which cross-reacts with the A and the B antigen. This explains the peculiar phenomena mentioned above.

Clinical significance of anti-C

This expanded version of the distribution of the naturally occurring iso-antibodies provides the most reasonable explanation for the well-known fact that group O mothers have babies affected with ABO haemolytic disease far more frequently than mothers of any other group. According to this view, it is the anti-C (in the Ig G form) in the serum of group O mothers which is responsible for the disease in the vast majority of cases. This problem is considered further in Chapter 13.

Sub-groups of A

All group A antigens are not identical. In fact, group A represents a heterogeneous collection of related antigens which have been called A_1, A_2, A_3, A_4 and A_5. From this it follows that all blood group As and ABs are not identical. For clinical purposes, only two of the sub-groups need be considered here—A_1 and A_2.

Group A_1 is distinguished from group A_2 by means of an antibody called anti-A_1. This antibody is regularly found in the serum of group B blood (together with anti-A) and sometimes in the serum of group A_2 and group A_2B blood. The reactions of A_1 and A_2 cells with anti-A and anti-A_1 are as follows.

Anti-A	Anti-A_1	
+	+	Sub-group A_1
+	−	Sub-group A_2

The nomenclature here causes difficulty to beginners. If the blood groups are called A_1 and A_2 why, they ask, are the antibodies not called anti-A_1 and anti-A_2. The fact is that the names given are not purely arbitrary but are based on the observed reactions. Anti-A is the comprehensive antibody which agglutinates all A cells. Anti-A_1 agglutinates only A_1 cells.

These simple reactions also illustrate another point which causes some difficulty—why a given blood specimen appears to have different blood group designations. In the above example, both specimens belong to group A, yet on further testing they are given two different designations, A_1 and A_2. The explanation is that 'A' is merely a family name, A_1 and A_2 are members of the family. It is important to grasp this simple point as similar difficulties occur in connection with the Rh system, but in this system the family relationships are not so obvious.

About 80 per cent of group A bloods are in fact group A_1 and about 20 per cent are A_2. The other weakly reacting members of the A family are rare.

There are two points of importance about the A_2 antigen. Firstly, it reacts more weakly than the A_1 antigen with anti-A serum. This is of little consequence in A_2 cells, but in A_2B cells the reaction may be so weak that it is overlooked. In this way an A_2B blood may be grouped as a B, and later transfused into a B patient. Special care must therefore be taken that the grouping serum used is capable of detecting the A_2 antigen in this combination. Secondly, A_2 and A_2B blood occasionally possess anti-A_1 in their sera. This irregularly occurring antibody would give rise to an incompatibility if A_1 or A_1B blood were used for transfusion.

The discovery of these sub-groups with their associated antibodies calls for a further extension of Table 1 given on page 8. See Table 5.

TABLE 5

Blood group	Antibodies regularly present	Antibodies sometimes present
A_1	anti-B	—
A_2	anti-B	anti-A_1
B	anti-A anti-A_1	—
A_1B	Nil	—
A_2B	Nil	anti-A_1
O	anti-A anti-A_1 anti-B anti-C	

RHESUS BLOOD GROUP SYSTEM

While the ABO blood group system is of primary importance in blood transfusion and of secondary importance in haemolytic disease of the newborn, the rhesus system is of importance in both. Almost 40 years elapsed between the discovery of the ABO and Rh systems. This is not surprising; the leaders in the field were busy extending their knowledge of the ABO system and discovering other systems such as the P and the MN. It was, in fact, while they were working on the MN system that Landsteiner and Wiener produced the antiserum by means of which the Rh system was discovered. This original antiserum was obtained by inoculating guinea-pigs with the red cells of a rhesus monkey. It is no longer used, being supplanted by better reagents obtained from human sources.

This anti-rhesus serum, now known as anti-Rh_0 (anti-D) divides the population into two groups—Rh positive and Rh negative.

Anti-Rh_0
(anti-D)
+ = Rhesus positive
− = Rhesus negative

Among people of European descent, some 85 per cent are Rh positive; the remaining 15 per cent are Rh negative.

Sub-groups of the Rh system

Subsequent to the discovery of anti-Rh_0, other rhesus antisera were discovered by means of which the rhesus system was subdivided into a great number of different types. Only two of these antisera, however, will be discussed here, anti-rh' and anti-rh". When Rh *positive* bloods are tested with these antisera, four different sets of reactions were obtained. Table 6 shows these reactions together with the symbols applied to the different sub-groups exposed by them.

TABLE 6

Anti-rh' (anti-C)	Anti-rh" (anti-E)		
+	−	=	Rh_1 (CDe)
−	+	=	Rh_2 (cDE)
−	−	=	Rh_0 (cDe)
+	+	=	Rh_z (CDE)

Similarly, when Rh *negative* bloods were tested with these two antisera, the four expected results were obtained (Table 7).

TABLE 7

Anti-rh' (anti-C)	Anti-rh" (anti-E)	
+	−	rh' (Cde)
−	+	rh" (cdE)
−	−	rh (cde)
+	+	rh_y (CdE)

Thus we see that there are four Rh positive and four Rh negative types.

Rhesus variants

The simple statement that the population is divided into Rh positive and Rh negative types requires some modification. Just as there are weakly reacting sub-groups of group A, so there are weakly reacting sub-groups of Rh. These weakly reacting Rh sub-groups, however, are not as well defined as the sub-groups of A and they are referred to collectively as Rh variant, or D^u. They differ not only from the standard Rh positive types but also from each other; some of them are so weakly reacting that they may appear, on testing, to be Rh negative.

They give negative reactions with Rh agglutinating serum but they absorb antibodies from incomplete Rh serum and in doing so they become Coombs positive. This is a practical laboratory means of distinguishing them from standard Rh positive and Rh negative types.

These Rh variants, having serological resemblances to both Rh positive and Rh negative red cells, cause considerable difficulty to clinicians as well as to serologists. For the purpose of blood donation they must be regarded as Rh positive because their antigen, though weak, may immunize an Rh negative recipient. For the same reason a husband who is Rh variant should be regarded as Rh positive. On the other hand, pregnant women and recipients of blood who are Rh variant, must be regarded as Rh negative because they are capable of being immunized by standard Rh positive blood.

Rhesus nomenclature

To express such a complicated blood group system by means of symbols must of necessity involve a complicated system of nomenclature. But further confusion is created by the existence of two rival

TABLE 8

CDE nomenclature		Rh nomenclature	
Written symbol	Spoken symbol	Written symbol	Spoken symbol
CDe	Big C, big D, little e	Rh_1	are aitch one
cDE	Little c, big D, big E	Rh_2	are aitch two
cDe	Little c, big D, little e	Rh_0	are aitch owe
CDE	Big C, big D, big E	Rh_z	are aitch zed
Cde	Big C, little d, little e	rh′	are aitch prime
cdE	Little c, little d, big E	rh″	are aitch double prime
cde	Little c, little d, little e	rh	are aitch
CdE	Big c, little d, big e	rh_y	are aitch why
D^u	D you	$\mathcal{R}$h	are aitch variant

systems of nomenclature, CDE and Rh, which are in common use. Let us therefore pause to consider and compare these two. In Table 5 the sub-groups already mentioned are listed in parallel in both systems together with the spoken form of each.

Points to note

(1) A big D in the CDE nomenclature and a big R in the Rh nomenclature indicates an Rh positive group.

(2) A little d in the CDE nomenclature and a little r in the Rh nomenclature indicates an Rh negative group.

(3) There is little to choose between the written symbols but the spoken symbol for the Rh nomenclature is much less cumbersome, indeed the CDE system is something of a tongue twister. Sometimes 'large' and 'small' are substituted for 'big' and 'little'—this worsens matters.

(4) The CDE system indicates the presence of a d antigen in all the Rh negative groups, yet, as there is no anti-d, this antigen has never been discovered.

(5) The CDE system shows more clearly than the Rh system, the antigens that are present on the cells. For example CDE tells us that antigens C, D, and E are present. In the corresponding Rh symbol we have to remember that Rh_z contains factors rh' and rh''. The alternative Rh symbol for Rh_z is Rh_1Rh_2 which is more expressive if slightly more cumbersome.

(6) D^u, in the CDE system, refers to a heterogenous collection of weakly reacting Rh positive red cells. But the symbol itself rather gives the impression of a single specific entity. Indeed certain antisera are labelled 'anti-D^u', a reagent which does not exist. The corresponding symbol in the Rh nomenclature is $\tilde{R}h$, a symbol which I can neither voice nor write. I therefore use the alternative Rh expression, 'Rh variant'. This is preferable also because it reminds us that we are referring to a variable group and not a specific entity.

(7) As the little h is common to all symbols in the Rh nomenclature for blood groups, some workers drop it thus making the Rh nomenclature even more concise. In this way Rh_1 becomes R_1, rh' becomes r'. This practice, however, may lead to confusion with Rh genes which are similarly indicated.

(8) The CDE system is more easy to learn than the Rh system.

MN BLOOD GROUP SYSTEM

The MN blood group system was discovered by the use of two

antisera, anti-M and anti-N, produced by injecting human red cells into rabbits. The reactions of these antisera are shown as follows.

Anti-M	Anti-N		
+	−	=	Group M
−	+	=	Group N
+	+	=	Group MN

It will be noted that, not four, but only three different kinds of reaction are found in this blood group system. There is thus no group corresponding to group O in the ABO system, or group Rh_0 in the Rh system. Because of this, the MN groups are particularly valuable in investigating cases of disputed parenthood.

The antigens are poorly antigenic in Man, and though M has been associated with both haemolytic disease of the newborn and incompatible blood transfusions, the events are so rare that this system is ignored in routine clinical work.

OTHER BLOOD GROUP SYSTEMS

Other blood group systems sometimes give rise to haemolytic disease of the newborn or blood transfusion reactions but these are rare. For ordinary transfusion purposes, blood banks group blood into the 4 ABO types and the 2 Rh types, thus giving eight types in all. This is all that is necessary for the vast majority of cases. Were the other blood group antigens to be taken into consideration, instead of these eight types, blood banks would have thousands of different types to deal with.

12—Immunology in blood transfusion

BLOOD TRANSFUSION

The first rule of blood transfusion is that the donor's red cells must not be given to any person who possesses antibodies which would react against them. The second rule is that the donor cells must not possess the Rh factor (the Rh_0 factor) if it is absent from the cells of the proposed recipient.

A glance at Table 1 on page 8 will show that, in so far as the ABO system is concerned, group A donor blood, for example, may not be given to a group O recipient. If it were given, the anti-A in the group O recipient's serum would react with the donor A cells and cause a serious, if not fatal, reaction. It will also be seen that a group O blood could be given (in terms of the first rule) to a group A recipient because such a recipient's serum does not possess any antibody which would react against the donor cells.

Cross transfusions

A point now arises which causes some difficulty. It might be thought that in the second example given above, the anti-A in the donor group O blood, would react with the recipient's A cells and that such a transfusion could therefore not be given. There is some merit in this thought, indeed it would be most unwise to give a massive transfusion of O blood to an A recipient for this very reason. But if the transfusion consisted of only one or two units (a unit is about 500 ml) the anti-A in the donor blood would be so diluted by the much larger volume of the recipient's blood, and it would be so neutralized by the group A substance in the recipient's plasma, that its effects would be negligible.

67

Fulfilment of the rules

To satisfy the requirement of Rule 1 and Rule 2, both donor and recipient must be grouped in regard to ABO and Rh, and a cross-matching test must be done using the recipient's serum and the donor's cells. It is important to remember that it is the cells of the donor which must not be attacked by the serum of the recipient.

Why group and cross-match?

As mentioned above, grouping and cross-matching are done to ensure that the requirements of both Rule 1 and Rule 2 are satisfied. Grouping alone is not sufficient because a group A donor blood, for example, might be quite incompatible with a group A patient's serum as a study of Table 5 on page 62 will show. Cross-matching alone is not sufficient because an Rh positive blood, for example, may be quite compatible with an Rh negative patient's serum. In fact, such a transfusion could be given with immediate good effect. But later, rhesus antibodies might develop and these could lead to complications. If the recipient were a young woman she might never be able to have a living child.

Time required for these tests

The methods commonly in use for grouping and cross-matching vary in detail from centre to centre. The grouping itself is a relatively short procedure, but at least one hour should be allowed for the standard Coombs cross-matching test. This is largely because of the prolonged incubation period which the test calls for (on average about 40 minutes). In case of emergency the time required for cross-matching can be reduced but only by sacrificing safety. This emergency method should therefore be requested only in cases of genuine emergency and not for convenience. Should a haemolytic reaction result from blood cross-matched in this way, the onus would be on the clinician to justify his request, and if he could not do so, he might have to face serious charges. In cases of desperate emergency, low titre group O blood (preferable Rh negative) may be administered without a cross-match.

It has often been suggested that every member of the community should be grouped so that, in the event of a transfusion being required, blood could be made available with less delay. As the delay, however, is due, not to the grouping, but to the cross-matching, it is questionable if such a scheme would be of any real value.

Cross-matching for newborn babies

Newborn babies have not yet developed their own iso-antibodies. Hence any antibodies in the baby's serum may be presumed to have passed to it from the mother. In cross-matching, therefore, it is usual to set the donor cells (which are of the baby's group) against the mother's serum. In those cases where the ABO groups are such that the baby could not be a donor for the mother, then the donor cells are cross-matched against the baby's serum.

In the usual cases of haemolytic disease of the newborn, Rh negative blood is selected for cross-matching even though the baby is Rh positive. Why? In cases of haemolytic disease of the newborn due to a rare antibody, the red cells of the mother may be used. It is preferable, in these cases, to suspend the mother's red cells in group AB serum.

High titre and low titre group O blood

The iso-antibody titre of group O blood varies considerably. Should it be above 200 it is considered high titre, while if it is below this figure it is considered low titre. High titre group O blood should be given to group O recipients only. Why? Low titre group O blood may be given to recipients of other ABO groups, provided the Rh groups correspond and provided a small transfusion only is given.

Universal donors and universal recipients

In the early days of blood transfusion these terms were in common use. Group O was the universal donor and group AB the universal recipient. From what has been said already, it will be apparent that strictly speaking there is no such thing as a universal donor and a universal recipient. Nevertheless, it must be said that few serious reactions will occur if group O low titre blood only were used for transfusion. In some countries, blood banks supply remote hospitals which have few or no laboratory facilities with such blood as a precaution against serious reactions.

Cross-matching

Very occasionally red cells fail to survive in the recipient despite a satisfactory compatibility *in vitro*. This underlines the point that the ultimate test for compatibility is the survival of the transfused cells in the recipient's circulation. Every transfusion therefore should be followed by a haemoglobin estimation of the recipient's blood and if the expected level is not obtained or maintained, the serum should be examined spectroscopically for the presence of methaemalbumen. In this way a hidden haemolytic transfusion reaction may be exposed.

Difficulties in cross-matching

Difficulties in cross-matching often arise in the laboratory because of the presence of an irregular antibody in the recipient's serum. A great variety of antibodies either alone or in combination may be present, the principal ones being anti-A_1, anti-Lewis, anti-P and anti-Rh. Sometimes difficulties arise due to excessive rouleaux. This was seen particularly if the recipient had had an infusion of Dextran shortly before his blood was collected for cross-matching. In such cases the laboratory should be informed that the Dextran infusion has been given. Adjustments can then be made and much time and effort saved.

Cross-matching in cases of autoimmune haemolytic anaemia

If the offending antibody is of the cold type, the difficulty in cross-matching can be overcome by carrying out every phase of the cross-matching test at 37°C. Subsequently, the donor blood and the patient should be kept warm during the transfusion. Great care should be taken when warming the donor blood. The container should not be held under a hot water tap, but immersed in a basin of warm water, the temperature of which ought to be checked with a thermometer. To over-heat blood is to invite a haemolytic reaction.

If the antibody is of the warm type, there may be difficulty not only in cross-matching but in grouping also. In fact, to group the cells of the patient, it may be necessary to elute any antibody which may have become attached to them. Such an attached antibody might block the antigen and thus make correct grouping impossible. Having established the group, donor cells of the same group are cross-matched against the patient's serum and against the eluate.

If the specificity of the offending antibody can be determined, then the magnitude of the problem will be seen, blood lacking the corresponding antigen may be fairly readily available, or it may be almost impossible to obtain. In these cases it is important to remember that a blood relative of the patient may be a suitable donor.

HAEMOLYTIC TRANSFUSION REACTIONS

Haemolytic transfusion reactions result from using the wrong blood, using time-expired blood, or using over-heated blood. The clinical manifestations vary greatly. They may be hardly perceptible—there may be pyrexia, rigors, and oliguria progressing to anuria, or there may be sudden collapse and death. In the average case, a raised temperature, rigors, jaundice and haemoglobinuria are the most prominent signs.

Management of a case

As soon as a haemolytic transfusion is suspected the transfusion must be discontinued. A fresh specimen of blood should be taken from the patient and this together with the remains of the donor blood (even if it is only a smear of blood on the walls of the container) should be returned to the laboratory. The patient should be put on a fluid intake-output chart and a specimen of his urine should be sent to the laboratory. All this should be done in every case without delay. From there on each case must be treated on its own merits and in the light of the laboratory results.

Immunological reactions other than haemolytic reactions

A variety of allergic reactions, urticaria, swelling of the face, erythematous rashes and even bronchial asthma, occur not infrequently during, or shortly after, a blood transfusion. These are attributed to an antigen in the donor blood to which the recipient is hypersensitive. Such incompatibilities cannot, of course, be detected in the laboratory.

In the majority of cases the attack is trivial but on occasions it may be quite severe, even alarming. They are usually readily controlled by adrenaline which should always be easily available.

Some practitioners, because of the frequency of these reactions, advocate the administration of antihistamines as a routine before all transfusions. Others say that the antihistamines should be given only to those patients who have a history of allergy; this seems more reasonable. In any event, the drugs should be given directly to the patient and not injected into the container of donor blood.

13—Immunology in materno-foetal incompatibility

As blood groups are genetically determined it follows that a baby's blood group is not necessarily the same as its mother's. If the materno-foetal blood groups are such that the baby could be a blood donor for the mother, then there is no materno-foetal incompatibility and the pregnancy is said to be homospecific. If, however, the materno-foetal blood groups are such that the baby could not be a donor for the mother, then there is a materno-foetal incompatibility and the pregnancy is regarded as heterospecific.

ABO MATERNO-FOETAL INCOMPATIBILITY

ABO materno-foetal incompatibility is very common. Fortunately, in the vast majority of cases it is of no serious consequence because the ABO iso-antibodies (usually of the Ig M type) cannot cross the placenta. Sometimes, however, placenta-passing Ig G antibodies appear in the mother's blood and in these cases the baby is liable to haemolytic disease of the newborn.

How common is ABO haemolytic disease?

It is quite impossible to answer this question in definite terms. There are those who say that in certain races it is more common, and therefore a greater community problem, than Rh haemolytic disease. Most authorities, however, say that it is much less common than Rh haemolytic disease and also that it is much less severe in the vast majority of cases.

Incidence of ABO haemolytic disease

A rather extraordinary situation arises in connection with ABO haemolytic disease in that one can often be quite categorical in saying

72

that it is *not* present as, for example, when the mother's blood group is A and the baby's blood group is O. Seldom, however, can one be categorical in saying that it *is* present. The situation is similar to that which arises in cases of disputed fatherhood—it is often possible to prove that the accused man is *not* the father, but never possible to prove that he *is*. In Table 9 are listed the various materno-foetal blood group combinations in which the disease may occur and also those in which it could not occur.

TABLE 9

ABO haemolytic disease possible		ABO haemolytic disease impossible	
Mother	Baby	Mother	Baby
O	A	O	O
O	B	A	O or A
A	B or AB	B	O or B
B	A or AB	AB	A, B, or AB

(Materno-foetal blood group combinations which permit and preclude the possibility of ABO haemolytic disease of the newborn.)

It will be noted that a group O baby cannot have ABO haemolytic disease and that a group AB mother cannot have a baby with ABO haemolytic disease. In practice, and for reasons mentioned on page 61, it will be found that in the vast majority of cases of ABO haemolytic disease the mother is group O and the baby either group A or group B. (Never AB. Why?)

A difficulty in diagnosis

ABO haemolytic disease may be so mild that it passes unnoticed or it may perhaps be mistaken for so-called physiological jaundice. Such mild cases and even moderate ones cannot be proved because the direct Coombs test, so valuable in Rh haemolytic disease, is of little value here as it usually gives negative results. In an endeavour to solve this problem Dunning modified the direct Coombs test by the use of a proteolytic enzyme. With this modified test Dunning found that ABO haemolytic disease occurs in some 80 per cent of the cases where it could possibly occur.

In view of these difficulties the only worthwhile advice that can be given is that newborn babies must be watched very carefully during the first 24 hours of life for the appearance of jaundice. This applies particularly if the mother is group O and the baby either group A or group B. If jaundice occurs, the bilirubin should be measured at frequent intervals and if the unconjugated bilirubin should approach

18 mg per cent the baby should be given an exchange transfusion.

RHESUS MATERNO-FOETAL INCOMPATABILITY

Rhesus haemolytic disease of the newborn arises when a woman who possesses placenta-passing Rh antibodies in her serum bears a child with the corresponding Rh antigen on its cells. In more than 95 per cent of cases the particular Rh antigen concerned is the one known as Rh_0 and the corresponding antibody is called anti-Rh_0.

How does a woman come to possess these antibodies?

These antibodies, like all other antibodies, arise as a result of stimulation by the corresponding antigen. Unlike the ABO iso-antibodies, however, they do not occur 'naturally'* but usually arise as a result of pregnancy when the mother is Rh negative and the baby Rh positive, or blood transfusion, when the recipient is Rh negative and the donor Rh positive. In the past, injections of blood were given for a variety of ailments and they were always given without prior grouping. This practice also resulted in the development of Rh antibodies in the recipient but fortunately it is now largely, if not completely, abandoned.

For practical purposes, therefore, it can be said that the presence of Rh antibodies in the serum of a woman indicates previous pregnancy or previous blood transfusion, while in the serum of a man they indicate previous blood transfusion. Of these two ways in which Rh antibodies arise, pregnancy is by far the more common, but transfusion is by far the more potent.

Incidence of rhesus haemolytic disease

Among people of European descent, some 85 per cent of the population are Rh positive and about 15 per cent are Rh negative. These proportions imply that in about 13 per cent of marriages the wife will be Rh negative and the husband Rh positive. This is the usual situation for the development of haemolytic disease of the newborn due to the Rh antigen and it accounts for more than 95 per cent of cases.

The disease, however, is by no means as common as this figure (13 per cent) might suggest. We must therefore look into the reasons for this fortunate deficiency of cases. The question may be considered under four headings.

(1) *Zygosity of the father*

About 50 per cent of men are heterozygous in regard to the Rh antigen. The other 50 per cent are homozygous. The chances of a

* There are rare exceptions.

heterozygous man having an Rh negative baby with an Rh negative woman is 50 per cent at each pregnancy. His entire family therefore of three or four children (a common number these days) could quite easily be Rh negative and therefore insusceptible to the disease. The children of the homozygous man will all, of course, be Rh positive.

(2) *Number of pregnancies*

The first child in an immunologically unfavourable marriage (wife Rh negative, husband Rh positive), even if it is Rh positive nearly always escapes the disease. This is because the antigenic stimulation of the mother occurs mainly during the birth of this child. There are therefore no antibodies developed for some days by which time the baby is born and thus out of danger. Future Rh positive babies cannot escape in this way.

(3) *Materno-foetal ABO situation*

If the materno-foetal ABO blood group situation is such that ABO haemolytic disease is possible (see Table 9, page 73) then there is a high degree of resistance to the development of Rh antibodies. This is because the baby's Rh positive (but ABO incompatible) cells are destroyed by the mother's ABO iso-antibodies before they can stimulate the development of Rh antibodies.

Arising out of this is the question of predicting the ABO group of the unborn baby. This can be achieved in some cases with accuracy by a consideration of the parents' ABO blood group (Table 10).

TABLE 10

Mother's ABO group	Father's ABO group	Baby's possible ABO group
O	A	O or A
O	B	O or B
O	AB	A or B
O	O	O
A	A	A or O
A	B	A, B, AB or O
A	AB	A, B, or AB
A	O	A or O
B	A	A, B, AB, or O
B	B	B or O
B	AB	B, A, or AB
B	O	B or O
AB	A	A, B, or AB
AB	B	B, A, or AB
AB	AB	A, B, or AB
AB	O	A or B

The prediction of the baby's ABO group from a consideration of the parent's ABO group. In only one combination can the baby's group be accurately predicted but this is a common combination (O × O). From this table we also see that materno-foetal incompatibility must exist when the mother is group O and the father group AB and that it never exists when the mother is group AB.

(4) *Immunologically unresponsive mothers*

Some Rh negative women, for unknown reasons, fail to develop Rh antibodies even though they may have borne Rh positive babies. The greater the number of Rh positive babies they bear, however, the greater their chances of developing such antibodies.

Rhesus haemolytic disease in other races

Among Negroid people and Indians the situation in regard to Rh incompatibility is more favourable than in people of European descent, because some 95 per cent are Rh positive and only 5 per cent Rh negative. These figures imply that an unfavourable rhesus mating would occur in only about 3 per cent of marriages. Furthermore, in Negroids, weak variants of the Rh antigen are far more common than in Europeans; hence antigenic stimulation of the mother is more commonly weaker and antigen-antibody reactions in the baby more commonly less avid.

Do rhesus antibodies really cause rhesus haemolytic disease?

The evidence collected in the last 25 years leaves no doubt that rhesus antibodies (of the Ig G type) are the primary cause of Rh haemolytic disease. Nevertheless, two kinds of observations have been made which preclude complacency in regard to the pathogenesis of the disease.

(1) Cases have been reported of twins of the same ABO and Rh groups being born, one severely and the other mildly (or hardly) affected by Rh haemolytic disease.

(2) The maternal titre of Rh antibodies is, broadly speaking, directly related to the severity of the disease in the baby. But there are exceptions. Thus, cases have been reported in which a high titre of maternal antibodies has been associated with a mildly affected baby— others have been reported in which a fairly low titre of maternal antibodies has been associated with a severely affected baby.

These observations show that there must be more to the pathogenesis of Rh haemolytic disease than just Rh antibodies. The final solution to this problem may provide a completely new method of treating the condition.

Immunological aspects of antenatal care

For practical purposes this subject resolves itself into the management of the Rh negative woman who is married to the Rh positive man. It is true that antibodies belonging to blood group systems other than the Rh system may be responsible for haemolytic disease of the newborn but these are either rare (Kell, MN, Duffy, Kidd) or relatively unimportant (ABO) and are dealt with after the birth of the baby as are those cases due to Rh antibodies other than anti-Rh_0. Different centres have slightly different routines but in all of them the objects of immunological care are as follows.

(1) To prevent the mother from being immunized against the Rh antigen. This is done shortly after birth in appropriate cases.

(2) To prevent the birth of a severely affected baby.

Principles of antenatal and postnatal care

To discuss this subject we will first consider the newly married woman who comes to the doctor for the first time in early pregnancy.

At the first visit a specimen of blood should be taken and grouped in regard to ABO and Rh. In addition, the serum should be examined for abnormal antibodies. If she is Rh positive, no further thought need be given to the immunological aspects of the case until the baby is born and then only if it shows signs of anaemia or jaundice. If she is Rh negative, her husband should be grouped also and if he, too, is Rh negative, then no further thought need be given until the birth of the baby.

If, however, he is Rh positive then the situation is correct for Rh immunization.* The husband may be tested to find out whether he is a homozygote or a heterozygote in regard to the Rh_0 factor. The information thus obtained may be a source of comfort (if he is a heterozygote) to the wife, but it will not influence the management of her case. An Rh negative woman who is pregnant by an Rh positive man, whether he be a homozygote or a heterozygote, must be considered a woman at risk and must be cared for accordingly.

If Rh antibodies are found in the mother's serum at this visit, it is reasonable to presume that they result from either a previous incompatible blood transfusion or a previous pregnancy. The former is likely to be admitted, the latter may well be denied. Irrespective of the origin of the antibodies, if the husband is Rh positive then the birth of an affected baby is to be expected and action must be taken accordingly.

Other abnormal antibodies which may be found in the mother's serum might cause bother should a transfusion be required at a later stage, so it is well to know about their existence in advance.

A rhesus negative primagravida with a rhesus positive husband

The patient may be assured that the chances of having an affected

* I am presuming that the husband of the wife is the father of the child, a presumption which does not always turn out to be correct.

baby are remote and that if it is affected it will not be a serious case. The main problem in this situation is to prevent Rh immunization of the mother and this is done after birth when the baby's Rh group is known.

Specimens of blood are taken from the patient at the 32nd and 38th week of pregnancy and examined for Rh antibodies. If antibodies are found, the birth of a mildly affected baby is to be expected. The pregnancy may be allowed to proceed normally unless the antibodies are of high titre. This is most unusual but when it does occur, induction of premature labour may be advisable.

Immediately after birth, the baby is grouped in regard to the Rh antigen. If it is Rh negative, no further action is called for. If, however, it is Rh positive the mother should be passively immunized against the Rh antigen to prevent active rhesus immunization.

Prevention of active rhesus immunization

The prevention of active Rh immunization is one of the major medical triumphs of the 1960s. Yet the principle of the method has been known since 1909 when Theobald Smith discovered that the induction of *passive* immunity in an animal against a given antigen would result in that animal being temporarily incapable of being *actively* immunized against the same antigen. The procedure consists in administering Rh antiserum to women at risk. The best-known serum at the present time is that prepared by Ortho laboratories, and marketed under the name of Rhogam, a name which indicates that it is a gamma globulin active against the all-important Rh factor, Rh_0. Rhogam administration is indicated in Rh negative women who give birth to Rh positive babies. If it is given within 72 hours of delivery it effectively destroys any of the foetal red cells which may have escaped into the maternal circulation. Thus, it prevents active maternal immunization. It should not be given to women who are already immunized against Rh_0 by, perhaps, a previous pregnancy or transfusion, and it should never, of course, be given to the baby. Why?

Reservations in the use of anti-rhesus immunoglobulin

Because of the world-wide shortage of anti-rhesus immunoglobulin at the present time the supply cannot meet the demand. It would seem fair, therefore, to limit its use to women to whom the following is applicable.

(1) Women who are not already immunized against the Rh antigen.

(2) Women with foetal (Rh positive) cells in their circulation as shown by microscopic examination of specially stained blood films.

(3) Women who, as far as the ABO blood groups are concerned, could be recipients of their babies' blood (homospecific pregnancies).

Rhesus negative multigravida with rhesus antibodies

A pregnant Rh negative woman with Rh antibodies represents what is perhaps the greatest problem facing the doctor. It requires much experience and the cooperation of obstetrician, paediatrician and immunologist to manage such cases successfully.

The crux of the problem is the Rh group of the baby. This, of course, is unknown and it is likely to remain unknown until the baby is born. If the father is found, on blood testing, to be probably homozygous, then a good guess can be made that the baby is Rh positive in which event it will be affected by Rh haemolytic disease. But if the father is found to be heterozygous, on which point definite information may be available, then there is a 50 per cent chance that the baby will be Rh negative and thus escape the disease.

The tests for the zygosity of the father therefore provide no definite information about the baby's Rh group other than the odds for or against it being Rh positive. For this reason it is questionable if they are worthwhile. One must therefore anticipate the worst—that the baby is Rh positive and that consequently it will be affected.

The next problem is to try to assess how badly the baby will be affected. This is done by the following procedure.

(1) The previous obstetrical history is considered.

(2) The Rh antibody titre is considered.

(3) The amniotic fluid is examined.

Charts, prepared by Liley in New Zealand and Freda in New York, are available to guide the practitioner in interpreting the results of amniotic fluid examination.

The final problem is to decide what action is to be taken should the evidence show that the baby *in utero* is affected. Intra-uterine transfusion is carried out in a few centres in the world but the greatest problem is if, and when, to induce labour. To induce premature labour is to remove the baby from its presumably harmful environment but it cannot be undertaken until the size of the baby justifies such action. On the other hand, to bring a premature baby into the world adds to the difficulties of the subsequent treatment. No general rule can be given for the solution of this dilemma. Each case must be treated on its own features and with regard to the facilities available.

A full appreciation of the problems outlined in this section is the greatest spur to the adoption of such preventive measures as were outlined in the previous one.

14—Autoallergic disease

DOMESTIC ANTIGENS

The whole idea of autoallergic disease is based on the fact that domestic antigens may, in violation of Ehrlich's theory of *horror autotoxicus*, become antigenic. That the body can produce antibodies reactive against its own tissue antigens can now no longer be doubted, but what is in doubt is the role of these antibodies in the pathogenesis of disease.

Before considering this question it is necessary to review the circumstances in which domestic antigens become antigenic. These may be considered under four headings.

(1) Alteration of domestic antigens.

(2) Cross-reactions.

(3) Late appearance of domestic antigens.

(4) Loss of control of antibody-producing apparatus.

Alteration of domestic antigens

A domestic antigen may be so altered by physical, chemical or infective means that it is in effect no longer a domestic antigen but a foreign antigen. It would then be recognized by the body as foreign and antibodies would be produced in the usual way. The alteration may take the form of exposing an antigenic chemical group which was previously hidden. This, as suggested by Dacie, may be what happens in certain haemolytic anaemias where antibodies with rhesus specificity have been found.

Viewed in this light, it could be said that as the domestic antigens were altered, the process is not truly autoallergic and that Ehrlich's principle was not violated.

Cross-reactions

It is easily possible that some pathogenic bacteria could possess antigens in common with certain tissues of the body. Infection with such bacteria could therefore lead to the production of antibodies which would cross-react with the antigens of these certain tissues. This process has been suggested as the cause of endocarditis following haemolytic streptococcal infection.

Such a mechanism, it might be argued, was also not a violation of Ehrlich's principle because it was the foreign antigens on the bacteria which stimulated the antibodies in the first place.

Late appearance of domestic antigens

Certain tissues, and therefore their antigens, develop long after immunological tolerance to other domestic antigens has been established. Such tissue antigens, therefore, though domestic, might be regarded as foreign by the antibody-producing apparatus. This mechanism has been invoked to explain some cases of male sterility.

Loss of control of antibody-producing apparatus

That the body so seldom produces antibodies reactive against domestic antigens shows that there must be control of some sort over its activities. That such a controlling mechanism would break down on occasions does not require a great feat of the imagination, even though the nature of the breakdown may be a complete mystery. For a variety of reasons, this seems to be the most common, but not the exclusive, means of autoallergy.

In terms of Jerne's theory of antibody production, it seems possible that the antibody-producing apparatus could, for some reason yet unknown, produce excess antibodies reactive against a particular tissue. In terms of Burnet's clonal selection theory, a clone of antibody-producing cells, which are normally forbidden, could emerge to produce antibodies reactive against a target tissue.

Effect of autoantibodies

Having seen possible ways in which autoantibodies may arise, we must now consider the effect of these antibodies on the tissues of the body. First, a few general remarks are required. Autoantibodies are found in a number of diseases the causes of which are unknown. Thus, rheumatoid arthritis, which in the past has been attributed to infection, allergy and stress, is now being attributed to autoantibodies. In support of this theory, the presence of autoantibodies, so often found in the sera of such cases, is cited. Identical antibodies, however, are often found in the sera of normal relatives of rheumatoid arthritis cases, and indeed, they are sometimes found even in the serum of normal blood donors.

The case, therefore, against autoantibodies in the pathogenesis of rheumatoid arthritis, is certainly not proven. Much the same can be said of Hashimoto's thyroiditis, systemic lupus erythematosus, pernicious anaemia, and other diseases now suspected of being autoallergic in origin.

The pathogenesis of haemolytic disease of the newborn is now well known and there is little doubt that iso-antibodies are the prime cause of it. A very similar disease occurs in adults in which autoantibodies become attached to the red cells and eventually lead to their premature destruction. As in haemolytic disease of the newborn, a few disturbing observations remain to be explained, but the consensus of informed opinion is that the autoantibodies cause the disease.

SPECIFIC DISEASES

Autoallergic haemolytic anaemia

After it was discovered that the direct Coombs test was positive in certain cases of haemolytic anaemia, it gradually came to be realized that these cases resulted from the action of autoantibodies. They were, therefore, called autoimmune or autoallergic haemolytic anaemias. A positive direct Coombs test is not in itself proof-positive of haemolytic anaemia as it is occasionally found in normal blood donors and others in whom there is no question of haemolytic anaemia. Having established the presence of haemolytic anaemia, however (by clinical, biochemical and morphological data), the presence of a positive direct Coombs test is sufficient evidence to regard it as autoallergic haemolytic anaemia. Such anaemias may occur in association with either warm or cold antibodies and are often classified accordingly.

Warm type

Autoallergic haemolytic anaemia of the warm type is the more common, being more than twice as common as the cold variety. The disease attacks all age groups, both sexes; it may be acute or chronic and apart from the general features of haemolytic anaemia, the patients present nothing by which the disease may be recognized at the bedside.

The blood picture shows the typical appearance of haemolytic anaemia, that is, a normochromic, normocytic regenerative anaemia, often with spherocytes. The bone marrow shows hyperplasia of the erythroid series as is expected in any case of haemolytic anaemia. The erythropoiesis is usually normoblastic in type but because of the excessive activity in the erythroid series, it may be megaloblastic.

A positive direct Coombs test marks the case as autoallergic in origin. Refinements of the Coombs test show that the cells may be coated with Ig G, Ig G and complement, or complement alone. When the antibody is of the Ig G type, it often shows rhesus specificity.

Irrespective of whether the Coombs test is positive by virtue of Ig G, Ig G and complement, or complement alone, the fundamental cause of the disease is unknown. In about half the cases there is an association with some other disease the most common of which are malignant lymphoma, lupus erythematosus and drug poisoning. In the other half there is no such association and the condition is referred to as idiopathic.

Cold type

Autoallergic haemolytic anaemia of the cold type is distinguished from the former by observing agglutination of the patient's red cells in the cold. A blood specimen, taken for routine blood count, is sometimes found to show marked agglutination by the time it reaches the laboratory. On warming the specimen, the agglutination disappears but returns again when the specimen cools. If the agglutination is slight it is not noticed in the specimen tube—it may be noticed when attempts are made to make a blood film, or subsequently when the film is examined microscopically.

The antibodies responsible for the condition are of the Ig M type and will be removed, as might be expected, from the cells by warming them to 37°C. But even at this temperature, complement will remain attached so that the cells will still give a positive direct Coombs test if the appropriate Coombs reagent is used.

Were it not for the fact that the skin temperature is often reduced to the level at which antibody activity occurs, this condition would hardly be a disease at all. The importance of keeping the patient warm is thus underlined. As in the warm type, about half the cases are associated with some other disease, principally atypical pneumonia and malignant lymphoma. The other half is idiopathic.

Hashimoto's disease

First described by Hashimoto in 1912, this disease manifests itself as a firm diffuse enlargement of the thyroid gland. It is often, but not always, associated with myxoedema. As regards thyroid function in these cases, the sequence of hyperthyroidism, euthyroidism, and hypothyroidism has been reported and it is suggested that this spectrum of thyroid activity may be associated with the same basic pathological process. Microscopic examination of the thyroid gland shows widespread destruction of the normal thyroid tissue which is replaced by a heavy infiltration of lymphocytes and fibrous tissue.

Thyroid antibodies

Antibodies reactive against some component of the thyroid gland, thyroglobulin, the second colloid antigen, and cytoplasmic microsomes, have been detected in a very high proportion of cases of Hashimoto's disease. The same, or similar, antibodies have been detected in cases of pernicious anaemia which is not altogether surprising as there is a well-known clinical association between pernicious anaemia and myxoedema. But what is surprising is that these antibodies have also been found in a significant number of normal blood donors. The case against autoantibodies as the cause of Hashimoto's disease is rather weak. This, however, does not exclude the possibility of autoallergy being concerned in the pathogenesis of the disease. The microscopic appearance of the gland is highly suggestive of delayed hypersensitivity.

Rheumatoid arthritis

The first point about rheumatoid arthritis is that it has a misleading name. True, the most prominent features of the disease in most cases are the joint lesions, but it also attacks the heart, the lungs, the blood vessels, the lymphatic glands, the gastro-intestinal tract, the kidneys, the eyes and the skin. So it is, like lupus erythematosus, a systemic or disseminated disease.

Evidence of an autoallergic basis

(1) Abnormal antibodies, mainly rheumatoid factor and antinuclear factor, are commonly found in the sera of rheumatoid arthritis cases. With improved techniques they may be found in all cases. They are, however, also found in some normal people.

(2) The characteristic lesion in rheumatoid arthritis is an infiltration of the synovial membrane with lymphocytes and plasma cells. This is similar to what occurs in Hashimoto's disease, homograft rejection, and classical cases of delayed hypersensitivity.

(3) There are similarities between rheumatoid arthritis and serum sickness which is a classical allergic, though not autoallergic, disease.

(4) Rheumatoid arthritis resembles lupus erythematosus for which there are strong autoallergic associations.

(5) No other suggested cause for rheumatoid arthritis has proved satisfactory.

(6) Drugs which suppress the immunological mechanism, such as corticosteroids, are of benefit to patients with rheumatoid arthritis.

Systemic lupus erythematosus

Until Hargraves described the LE cell, it was generally considered that lupus erythematosus was a skin disease and nothing more. But with this discovery it gradually came to be realized that the same pathological process was the basis of a great many and varied sicknesses. Today, therefore, it is recognized that lupus erythematosus attacks the heart, the pleurae, the joints, the kidneys, the blood, the spleen, the liver, the lymphatic glands and the skin. All this leads to a multiplicity of clinical features which often mislead the practitioner, indeed lupus erythematosus now holds the title of the great masquerader, a title formerly held by syphilis. In fact, the masquerade may be so complete that even the Wasserman reaction may be positive.

Evidence of an autoallergic basis

(1) The LE phenomenon (see page 95).

(2) The presence of antinuclear factor (see page 96).

(3) The clinical similarity between lupus erythematosus and rheumatoid arthritis.

(4) The clinical observation that drugs which suppress the immunological mechanism, such as corticosteroids, are of great benefit to patients with lupus erythematosus.

(5) The fact that no other satisfactory cause has ever been found.

Despite the abundance of autoantibodies in this condition, there is no direct correlation between their presence and the activity of the disease. There is evidence of a delayed hypersensitivity reaction in some cases as is shown by the lymphocyte transfer test.

Pernicious anaemia

For many years pernicious anaemia was regarded primarily as a disease of the stomach characterized morphologically by varying degrees of gastritis, and functionally by an absence of intrinsic factor. About 10 years ago, however, Taylor and Schwartz showed that the serum of patients with pernicious anaemia had the ability to block the absorption of vitamin B_{12} when fed to other patients with pernicious anaemia. This extraordinary phenomenon was attributed to an antibody in the serum reactive against intrinsic factor.

The antibody is almost always absent in cases of gastritis unassociated with pernicious anaemia, but it is present in only a little more than half the patients with the disease. And it seems to make no difference to the patient whether it is absent or present. Its role, therefore, in the pathogenesis of pernicious anaemia is very doubtful.

Subsequently another antibody, reactive against the parietal cells of the gastric mucous membrane, was discovered in cases of pernicious anaemia. It is present in some 80 per cent of cases, but it is also present in a considerable number of patients with other diseases, including Hashimoto's disease, and also in a considerable number of normal people. So once again, the case against antibodies is far from conclusive.

That delayed hypersensitivity might be involved in the pathogenesis of pernicious anaemia is suggested by the close microscopical resemblance between the stomach in pernicious anaemia, the thyroid gland in Hashimoto's disease, and the classical examples of delayed hypersensitivity.

Ulcerative colitis

This disease is characterized by an intense inflammation and ulceration of the mucous membrane of the colon. The entire colon may be affected. Like pernicious anaemia, it is, in its natural history, subject to remissions and relapses.

For many years the aetiology of the condition was unknown. Infection, of course, was suggested and although it undoubtedly plays a part in the evolution of the disease, it hardly initiates the process. Then, for a long time, emotional stress was considered to be an important factor in the pathogenesis.

In 1959, Broberger and Perlman demonstrated the presence of abnormal antibodies in the serum of a high proportion of patients with the disease. These antibodies were reactive against human foetal colon and this was the first suggestion of an autoallergic process in the pathogenesis. But as so often happens, the case against the antibodies was far from conclusive.

Subsequently the same workers discovered that leucocytes from patients with ulcerative colitis were cytotoxic for the cells of foetal colon in tissue culture. This suggested delayed hypersensitivity as a possible mechanism in the pathogenesis. This view was supported by the observations that some patients with ulcerative colitis gave a positive result in the lymphocyte transfer test. Furthermore, the microscopic appearance of the mucous membrane in ulcerative colitis is not inconsistent with that of delayed hypersensitivity. The ulceration, leading inevitably to secondary infection, however, obscures what might otherwise be the classical picture.

15—Immunology in the diagnosis of disease

BASIC IMMUNOLOGICAL RESPONSES

We have seen previously that there are three basic immunological responses. The demonstration of the presence of one or other of these is used in the diagnosis of a variety of infectious and non-infectious diseases—thus, the demonstration of the following.

(1) Type 1 responses (circulating antibodies) are used in the diagnosis of typhoid fever, typhus fever, brucellosis, infective mononucleosis, leptospirosis, gonorrhoea, syphilis and various virus infections.

(2) Type 2 responses (immediate hypersensitivity) are used in the diagnosis of hydatid disease, trichinosis, filariasis, schistosomiasis, as well as the various allergic conditions discussed in Chapter 8.

(3) Type 3 responses (delayed hypersensitivity) are used for the diagnosis of tuberculosis, leprosy, brucellosis, dermatomycosis, coccidiomycosis, histoplasmosis and other fungal diseases.

General remarks

Because of the great number of serological tests available, and because of the difficulty in interpreting them in some cases, it cannot be stressed too often that in order to get the best service from the laboratory, cooperation between clinician and pathologist is required. In the experience of most laboratory workers, only clinicians who have themselves worked in a laboratory fully appreciate this. Cooperation includes collecting the correct specimen at the correct time and in the correct container. It includes submitting a short relevant history of the case and it includes a discussion between clinician and pathologist should unexpected results be reported.

Every practitioner, therefore, would do well to visit his local laboratory, make himself acquainted with the service it offers and its requirements in regard to the collection of specimens. Pathologists usually welcome such an approach.

SEROLOGICAL TESTS IN THE DIAGNOSIS OF DISEASE

Here we will discuss various tests commonly used in the diagnosis of disease. It must be remembered, however, that different laboratories may use different tests or different modifications of the same basic test. The results obtained from one laboratory, therefore, may not be quite the same as those obtained from another. Serological tests fall generally into one of four groups—agglutination tests, precipitation tests, complement-fixation tests, and haemagglutination-inhibition tests.

Enteric fever

The Widal test is the agglutination test used in the diagnosis of enteric fever. The test detects and measures the strength of circulating antibodies reactive against the antigens on the bacilli of typhoid and closely related organisms. In the United Kingdom the usual antigens used are the O and H antigens of Salm. typhi and Salm. paratyphi B because of the predominance of typhoid and paratyphoid B infection. In addition, a common non-specific H antigen is used. In other areas of the world, the antigens of other organisms are used, for example, those of Salm. paratyphi C.

The results of the test are expressed as the highest dilution (or titre) of the serum which gives agglutination. Far more important than a high titre is a rising titre, especially a rising O titre. Nevertheless, in a person who has not been vaccinated against enteric fever, an O titre of 100 or an H titre of 50 during the first ten days or so of a fever, is highly suggestive. The test should be repeated within a week to discover if the titres are rising.

The principle of this test can be used to recognize the Vi antigen. Antibodies reactive against the Vi antigen are of no great significance in the diagnosis of cases but are valuable in detecting carriers.

Salmonella food poisoning

The principle of the Widal test is employed in the retrospective, but not in the immediate, diagnosis of Salmonella food poisoning. The immediate laboratory diagnosis depends on culturing the organism.

Brucellosis

The same principle as in the Widal test is employed in the diagnosis of brucellosis, but the interpretation is even more difficult. Positive cases show titres of anything from 500 to 2,500. A negative result, however, does not exclude the disease. As in the Widal, a rising titre is more important than a high titre. If agglutination tests are negative, it is common practice in some laboratories to do a brucella Coombs test.

Gonorrhoea

The gonococcal complement-fixation test (GCFT) is the only serological test available for the diagnosis of gonorrhoea. Unfortunately, it gives false negative results in a very high percentage of cases, especially cases of early infection. For such cases, therefore, it must be stressed that the laboratory diagnosis of gonorrhoea depends on the direct identification of the organism in a smear made from the pus, or less commonly, by culturing the organism from the pus. Positive results with the GCFT, however, are significant and are of value in the diagnosis of chronic gonorrhoea, especially chronic salpingitis.

Syphilis

A great number of serological tests have been devised for the diagnosis of syphilis. This fact in itself is proof that none of them is completely satisfactory. Among the most commonly used are complement-fixation tests (the Wasserman and its various modifications, and the Reiter protein complement-fixation test) and a variety of precipitation tests (Kahn, Meinicke, Ide, Eagle, Price and VDRL).

None of these tests is specific; I once made a list of some 40 diseases which are known to be associated with a positive Wasserman reaction. Nor are they all equally sensitive. Where, then, does the practitioner stand in regard to the serological diagnosis of syphilis? It is usual practice to do both a Wasserman test and one or other of the precipitation tests. Which of the precipitation tests is done will depend on the laboratory to which the specimen is sent. If there is a disparity in the results, the laboratory will usually pursue the matter further and report accordingly. Furthermore, if positive, the laboratory will do a quantitative test (usually a quantitative Wasserman) in order to establish a base line from which the effects of treatment may be assessed.

Interpretation

This is often difficult. On the sole basis of positive serological tests, many a patient has been subjected to the treatment (not to mention the stigma) of syphilis, who was, in fact, suffering from glandular fever or malaria. If the tests are done in a routine (army recruits, blood donors, pregnant women) and found to be positive, and if there is definite clinical evidence of syphilis, then treatment may be started. If, however, there is no definite evidence of syphilis, then the tests should be repeated. If they are still positive then the treponema immobilization test should be done. This test becomes positive later than the others but even it is not completely specific for syphilis. Nevertheless, it is generally regarded as the final court of serological appeal.

If the clinical evidence suggests the diagnosis of syphilis and if the preliminary serological tests are negative, again the tests should be repeated and, if necessary, they should be repeated in another laboratory. If the tests from one laboratory differ from those of another, the pathologists from both laboratories should be informed. This, contrary to general opinion, will be a source of pleasure rather than embarrassment.

Positive serological tests in the newborn infant of an affected mother do not necessarily mean that the child has syphilis. The antibodies responsible for the positive results may have passed across the placenta from mother to baby. Such a case, however, would arouse the greatest suspicion. Quantitative tests will show a rapidly falling titre if, in fact, the baby is not infected.

Leptospirosis

The term leptospirosis includes Weil's disease and canicola fever. Circulating antibodies can usually be detected after the first week of the disease and appropriate agglutination tests can distinguish between L. icterohaemorrhagiae and L. canicola. Once again, the importance of a rising titre is stressed but any doubtful result should be discussed with the pathologist. During the first week, if the disease is suspected, the blood should be examined for leptospires.

Typhus fever

Although typhus fever is caused by organisms of the rickettsia group, the serum of a person with this disease will agglutinate in high titre completely unrelated organisms—namely one or other of the proteus group of bacteria. This is because the two organisms, rickettsia and proteus, have antigens in common. The test is commonly known as the Weil-Felix test. The particular strain of proteus organism used depends on the kind of typhus sought and this will vary in different parts of the world. Commonly, proteus OX 19 and proteus OX K are used. Titres of 50 are suggestive but, as before, a rising titre is the most significant finding. As cross-reactions are common, it is very likely that the pathologist will have to be consulted to help interpret positive results.

Glandular fever (infective mononucleosis)

Paul-Bunnell test

Most normal sera possess antibodies which will agglutinate sheep cells. These naturally occurring antibodies are of the Forssman type and can be absorbed from the sera by means of a suspension of guinea-pig kidney. The sera of many patients with glandular fever will agglutinate sheep cells and in very high dilution. Furthermore, these antibodies are not absorbed from the serum by guinea-pig kidney. That is the basis of the Paul-Bunnell test for glandular fever.

A difficulty arises because the serum of persons who have had serum sickness may also agglutinate sheep cells in high dilution. The antibodies responsible for this reaction are absorbed from the serum by ox cells and by guinea-pig kidney. In this way the difficulty is overcome.

To summarize, it seems that there are three different kinds of antibody to be considered in connection with the Paul-Bunnell test.

(1) The naturally occurring Forssman type antibody which is absorbed by guinea-pig kidney but not by ox cells.

(2) The glandular fever antibody which is not absorbed by guinea-pig kidney but which is absorbed by ox cells.

(3) The serum sickness antibody which is absorbed by both guinea-pig kidney and by ox cells.*

In the full, or differential, Paul-Bunnell test, therefore, the patient's serum is titrated against sheep cells without absorption and after absorption with both guinea-pig kidney and ox cells. The test often becomes positive during the first week of the disease but sometimes it is delayed for three to six weeks and sometimes it never becomes positive. That the serum of some patients do not give positive results is probably because at least two different viruses may cause the disease.

* In fact other antibodies have been discovered in the serum of glandular fever cases, one is reactive against the EB virus of Burkitt's lymphoma, the other, sometimes present, gives a positive Wasserman reaction.

'Denco-I.M. test'

The 'Denco-I.M. test' is a simple and reliable test for glandular fever which is particularly useful when only occasional testing is required. In this test a drop of 4 per cent horse cells is mixed with a drop of patient's serum on a clean glass slide. A positive result is shown by agglutination of the cells which often occurs in a matter of a few seconds. No agglutination within two minutes indicates a negative reaction.

OTHER VIRUS INFECTIONS

There are complement-fixation tests available for psittacosis, Q fever, and lymphogranuloma venereum. Influenza and mumps antibodies may be detected either by complement-fixation or haemagglutinin-inhibition tests. The discovery of a rising titre of mumps antibodies will help in the diagnosis of those atypical cases of mumps in which there is little or no enlargement of the parotid glands. Serological tests play little part in the diagnosis of smallpox.

There is an urgent need for reliable serological tests for infective hepatitis and homologous serum jaundice.

Amoebiasis

Once considered to be a disease of the intestines and the tropics, amoebiasis is now known to be widely distributed outside both. It is a difficult disease to recognize and may be confused with a great many other diseases including cirrhosis of the liver, pyogenic liver abscess, infective hepatitis, lobar pneumonia, pulmonary tuberculosis, bacillary dysentery, typhoid fever and others.

Examination of the stool for the cysts or vegetative forms of *entaboeba histolyticum* is the time-honoured method but this is difficult (I know of no parasite in the stool more difficult to recognize than *entamoeba histolyticum*) and therefore not satisfactory. Among the serological tests for amoebiasis the following seem to be the most commonly used.

(1) *Complement-fixation test*

Complement-fixation tests for this disease are available in centres throughout the world. Opinions of their value vary greatly, this is probably because the antigens used in the test also vary greatly. Many workers report that while it is a reliable test in cases of amoebic liver abscess, it is unreliable in cases of amoebic dysentery.

(2) *Gel-diffusion test (Ouchterlony technique)*
Powell (1969) summarizes his experience with the gel-diffusion test as shown in Table 11.

TABLE 11

	Number of patients	Percentage positive
Amoebic dysentery	718	94
Amoebic liver abscess	753	98
Symptomless cyst passers	96	34
Other diseases (African)	710	14
Other diseases (Indian)	174	4
Other diseases (European)	136	0

These figures speak for themselves. In particular, it should be noted that a high degree of sensitivity is combined with a high degree of specificity. Powell stresses that the correct interpretation of the results calls for a knowledge of the serological status of the population under consideration. Thus a positive gel-diffusion test in an African living in Durban would not be as significant as that of a European living in Durban. Why?

Lupus erythematosus

A number of serological tests may give positive results in cases of systemic lupus erythematosus and this might well lead to further confusion of a problem which is already likely to be confused from the clinical aspects of the case. Thus, the rheumatoid factor has been reported positive in some 50 per cent of cases of lupus erythematosus, the direct Coombs test and the Wasserman reaction are often positive, and antibodies reactive against white blood cells and platelets are present in up to 80 per cent of cases.

Small wonder, therefore, that the clinician gets lost in a welter of positive serological results. The above-mentioned tests should be done where indicated, not for the purpose of putting a label on the case but in order to achieve an assessment of the patient as a whole.

The serological features of lupus erythematosus should be studied in conjunction with those of rheumatoid arthritis which it resembles so closely. The tests most generally used for the diagnosis of lupus erythematosus are as follows.

(1) *Demonstration of the LE phenomenon*
Until recently this was the most commonly used test for the diagnosis of lupus erythematosus. The phenomenon, which was first

described by Hargraves, consists of a phagocyte, usually a neutrophil, sometimes a monocyte, which contains a rounded mass of degenerated nuclear material in its cytoplasm. The mass, which is homogeneous and basophilic, is so bulky that it displaces the nucleus of the phagocyte peripherally and seems to press it against the cell wall. The whole appearance is characteristic and is called the LE cell.

The factor responsible for this phenomenon is an immunoglobulin G which has antibody activity reactive against desoxyribonucleoprotein. The LE cells are seen in some 80 per cent of cases of lupus erythematosus but as they occur in other conditions also (up to 30 per cent of cases of rheumatoid arthritis) they are not pathognomonic of this condition. Nevertheless, as it is a comparatively simple, if tedious test to do, it should be done in all suggestive cases of lupus erythematosus.

(2) *Demonstration of antinuclear factor by immunofluorescence*
This is the most valuable test for lupus erythematosus at the present time. It is positive in almost all cases. Antinuclear factors are also found in rheumatoid arthritis but in this condition heat-labile immunoglobulin M antibodies, which give a speckled appearance in the immunofluorescence test are detected; in lupus erythematosus they are mainly heat-stable immunoglobulin G antibodies which give a homogeneous fluorescence. This distinction is fine and certainly cannot be made by the occasional performer.

Rheumatoid arthritis

The first point about rheumatoid arthritis is that it has a misleading name. True, the most prominent features of the disease in most cases are the joint lesions, but it also affects the heart, the lungs, the blood vessels, the lymphatic glands, the gastro-intestinal tract, the eye, the skin and subcutaneous tissue and the blood. So it is, like lupus erythematosus, a systemic or disseminated disease.

It is little wonder, therefore, that it is often a difficult disease to recognize and that recourse is often made to the laboratory. Some 80 per cent of cases of rheumatoid arthritis possess a protein in their sera called rheumatoid factor. This protein is in fact an antibody which reacts with gamma globulin. It is thus an anti-gamma globulin and its demonstration forms the basis of two commonly used tests for rheumatoid arthritis.

(1) *Rose-Waaler test*
In this test, red cells coated with gamma globulin are mixed with the patient's serum. If the patient's serum possesses the rheumatoid factor, the cells will agglutinate.

(2) *Latex fixation test*

In this test, polystyrene latex particles are substituted for the red blood cells as described above in the Rose-Waaler test. The latex particles are coated with gamma globulin and they agglutinate when mixed with the patient's serum if that serum contains the rheumatoid factor. This test is conveniently done by means of a kit supplied by Hyland Laboratories.

Interpretation

Although they do not give absolutely parallel results there is little to choose between the two tests. Nevertheless, it is probably good practice to do both in suspected cases. They are positive in about 80 per cent of cases of rheumatoid arthritis but they give negative results in a few indubitable cases of this disease. A negative result, therefore, does not exclude rheumatoid arthritis. They also give positive results in Still's disease and in lupus erythematosus but they are negative in osteoarthritis, acute rheumatic fever, ankylosing spondylitis and infective arthritis, any of which might be mistaken for rheumatoid arthritis.

Hashimoto's disease

Three distinct kinds of antibody are found in the sera of patients with Hashimoto's disease. These are reactive against three corresponding components of the thyroid gland—namely thyroglobulin, the so-called second antigen of the colloid, and the microsomal antigen.

All three of these antibodies can be detected by the immunofluorescence technique of Coons, but, in addition, the Ouchterlony technique, the tanned cell technique and the latex particle agglutination technique can be used to detect thyroglobulin antibodies, while a complement-fixation test has been devised for the microsomal antibodies.

As these antibodies are found in the serum of persons with other diseases and even in that of some normal persons, their demonstration is of limited value in diagnosis. It is, however, useful in those cases of Hashimoto's disease where it is necessary to distinguish this condition from simple, and especially from malignant, goitre. The result of such serological tests, however, should be discussed with the serologist and confirmed by biopsy.

Infertility

A small proportion of cases of infertility, estimated at about 10 per cent are due to immunological factors. In these cases the serum of the wife contains antibodies reactive against the spermatozoa of the husband. The presence of these antibodies can be identified by a modified agglutination test using the wife's serum and the husband's spermatozoa.

Pregnancy

Although pregnancy is hardly a disease, it is included here because serological methods for its recognition are now replacing the older biological methods, such as the Aschheim-Zondek test, the Friedman test and the Hogben test. All these biological methods depended upon the demonstration of chorionic gonadotrophin. When, however, specific antibodies reactive against this protein hormone were discovered, several serological tests became feasible.

In one technique, rabbits are injected with purified gonadotrophin and in due course they produce anti-gonadotrophin antibodies. The serum of such rabbits provide the antibody required for the test. Sheep cells coated with human chorionic gonadotrophin provide the antigen. When these two reagents are mixed together agglutination of the sheep cells occurs. If, however, the urine of a pregnant woman is first added to the antiserum, the agglutination is inhibited and this constitutes a positive result.

A similar test uses latex particles coated with human chorionic gonadotrophin instead of sheep red blood cells. It gives parallel results. Once the reagents are prepared the tests take only a few minutes to complete and are very reliable.

Hydatid disease (echinococcus disease)

The Casoni test consists of an intradermal injection of antigen prepared from hydatid cyst fluid. That obtained from oxen, sheep and pigs is used. A positive result is shown by the appearance of a weal surrounded by an area of erythema at the site of injection. There may, or may not be, pseudopodia. The weal appears within 15 minutes, often within 10 minutes, and is a typical example of an immediate hypersensitivity reaction. Occasionally, a delayed reaction occurs. The test is reasonably reliable but sometimes both false negative and false positive results are given.

Trichinosis (trichina spiralis disease)

The Bachman test consists of an intradermal injection of antigens prepared from trichinae. This preparation is sometimes called trichinellin. As in the Casoni test, a positive reaction is shown by the immediate appearance of a weal at the site of injection. The test is reasonably reliable and becomes positive after the second week of the disease.

Filariasis (wucheria bancrofti disease)

In this test, the antigen consists of a saline extract of the organisms which is injected intradermally. The immediate appearance of a weal is a fairly reliable indication of the presence of the disease. More reliable, of course, is the demonstration of the parasites in the blood.

Schistosomiasis

The antigen consists of an alcoholic extract of infected snails' livers. It is injected intradermally. The immediate appearance of a weal is a reasonably good indication of infection. The urine and the stools, however, should be examined microscopically for ova.

Brucellosis

The antigen, which is injected intradermally, consists either of a diluted brucella vaccine, or a special preparation made for diagnostic purposes. A positive result is shown by an area of erythema and induration after 24 to 48 hours. This indicates past or present infection. As this test may well stimulate antibody production, the brucella agglutination tests should be done first.

Tuberculosis

The Mantoux test, of which there are several modifications, consists in the intradermal injection of purified protein derivative of mycobacterium tuberculosis. A positive result is shown by the appearance of an area of erythema and induration at the site of injection within 24 to 48 hours. Positive results indicate past or present infection.

This test is the classical example of delayed hypersensitivity occurring in the skin; it is discussed more fully on page 47.

Leprosy

The antigen, which consists of a suspension of leprosy tissue and which is sometimes called lepromin, is injected intradermally. A delayed reaction, as in the Mantoux test, is the positive result and is said to be reasonably reliable.

Lymphogranuloma inguinale

In the Frei test, the antigen formerly used consisted of material prepared from an infected lesion. This was injected intradermally. In more recent times the antigen used is a suspension of killed lymphogranuloma inguinale viruses. A positive result is shown by an area of erythema which appears within 24 to 48 hours.

Histoplasmosis

The antigen used is a culture filtrate of histoplasma capsulatum and is commonly called histoplasmin; 0·1 ml, in various dilutions, is injected intradermally. A positive reaction is shown by the appearance of a typical delayed hypersensitivity response.

Coccidioidomycosis

The antigen, known as coccidioidin, is a culture filtrate of C. immitis; 0·1 ml of various dilutions is injected intradermally. As in the previous test, a positive reaction is shown by a typical delayed hypersensitivity reaction.

Sarcoidosis

The Kveim test consists of an intradermal injection of sarcoid lymph gland tissue. A positive result is shown by the appearance of a papule at the site of injection within six weeks, sometimes within four weeks. Microscopic examination of the papule shows the typical appearance of sarcoid.

Schick test

The Schick test is a test, not for diphtheria, but for susceptibility to diphtheria. The antigen consists of diphtheria toxin 0·1 of which is injected intradermally. A positive result, indicating susceptibility to diphtheria, is shown by the appearance of an area of erythema and induration at the site of injection in 24 to 36 hours. A negative reaction indicates insusceptibility to diphtheria.

16—Immunology in the prevention of disease

THREE GROUPS OF INFECTIONS

The prevention of disease was the initial great promise of immunology and it was this that gave impetus to the growth of the science. In some instances this promise has been fulfilled, in some it has been partly fulfilled and in some it has not been fulfilled at all. The situation in regard to the value of immunological methods in the prevention of disease at the present time may be summarized by dividing the infections into three groups—A, B and C.

Group A

Group A infections are the infections for which there is a reasonably safe and effective vaccine available. The members of this group are smallpox, yellow fever, poliomyelitis, measles, rubella, typhus, tetanus, diphtheria, whooping cough, typhoid fever, tuberculosis and anthrax.

Group B

Group B infections are the infections for which vaccines are available but which, for one reason or another, the vaccines are unsatisfactory. They include the common cold, influenza, cholera, leprosy and plague.

Group C

Group C infections are the infections for which there is urgent need for a safe and effective vaccine. In addition to those mentioned in group B they include infective hepatitis, homologous serum jaundice, syphilis, gonorrhoea, cerebrospinal fever, dysentery, and infections due to streptococci, staphylococci, and the parasites.

ASSESSMENT OF VALUE OF VACCINATION

It must be remembered that it is difficult to assess the efficacy of a procedure which aims at protecting against the occurrence of an irregularly occurring event. In the natural course of things only a proportion (and sometimes only a small proportion) of a community at risk actually contracts the disease for which immunization is recommended. Furthermore, other factors militating against the disease in question may come into operation. Since the introduction of vaccination against typhoid fever, for example, there has been a great decrease in the incidence of that disease. But in this period also, there has been a great improvement in the standard of hygiene and nutrition. This doubtlessly contributed in large measure to the declining incidence of typhoid fever. Hence, vaccination may get credit which it does not deserve.

Conversely, vaccination against a specific disease may fail in certain cases through no fault of the basic immunological idea. The procedure may have been wrongly performed, performed too late in the course of an epidemic, performed using an impotent vaccine, or performed using the wrong strain of organism. Thus, the procedure may also receive adverse criticism which it does not deserve.

MATERIALS USED FOR VACCINATION

The word 'vaccination' is derived from the Latin word *vacca* meaning a cow; it was originally used in connection with Jenner's material but nowadays it is used to denote any material used deliberately to induce immunity. The material used for vaccination falls into three classes—dead bacteria and viruses, live but attenuated organisms, and toxoids.

Dead bacteria and viruses

Dead bacteria and viruses are used for a number of bacterial and virus infections. Although effective, they are generally not as effective as live vaccines. They are, however, safer. The method of killing the organisms varies—heat, formalin, phenol, alcohol and ultra-violet radiation have all been used. TAB is a typical example of a dead bacterial vaccine.

Live attenuated organisms

Live attenuated organisms are also extensively used. They generally produce a much better degree of immunity, but they are more dangerous. Typical examples of diseases for which live vaccines are used include tuberculosis and smallpox.

Toxoids

Toxoids are toxins which have been rendered non-toxic by treatment with formalin. Though non-toxic, they retain their antigenic properties. They are used mainly to produce immunity against diphtheria and tetanus.

VACCINATION ROUTINE

There is a tendency to believe that as vaccination is now a well-established practice, there is no need to change a routine which has been in use for perhaps decades. Further thought, however, will show that this belief is unfounded and that vaccination routines should indeed be revised from time to time. The following are the considerations which lead to this view.

(1) No vaccine is 100 per cent safe. The dangers of vaccination, therefore, must be weighed against the risks of not vaccinating. Thus to vaccinate a person who lives in London against yellow fever is not justified, but to vaccinate a person who lives in West Africa against yellow fever is perfectly justified. Similarly, in countries which have been free or almost free from smallpox for a number of years, vaccination against smallpox is not urgent. This, of course, is not an excuse for complacency.

(2) The times of vaccination and re-vaccination should be revised periodically depending on the risk of contracting the disease against which the vaccine is used, and also on the priorities of vaccination against other diseases. Such priorities change from time to time. In the United Kingdom, for example, smallpox vaccination may be deferred until immunity against diphtheria, whooping cough and measles has been established.

(3) New and improved vaccines appear on the market from time to time, hence a vaccine which was the most effective and the safest five years ago may not be the most effective or safest at the present time.

(4) Population migrations may lead to a situation where vaccination or re-vaccination is required at short notice. With the advantages of modern air-travel comes the disadvantage that no country is safe from an outbreak of an unexpected disease. A person incubating smallpox may board an aircraft in Calcutta, and in a few hours he may be in London.

For these reasons there can be no fixed vaccination routine. Even during the preparation of this book changes were made in the vaccination routine for certain diseases in the United Kingdom. It therefore behoves the practitioner to make himself acquainted with the latest official recommendations in the region in which he is in practice. Health authorities usually issue pamphlets or booklets recommending vaccination schedules which are currently applicable in their respective countries.

Immunity in the newborn

A newborn baby is unable to make its own gamma globulin and therefore its own antibodies. This inability persists for some six weeks. Hence, we must enquire into the means by which it is protected during this period.

Fortunately the human placenta (but not that of all animals) is capable of transmitting antibodies from the mother's blood to that of the foetus. In this way the baby is born with the same concentration of antibodies in its blood as the mother. Thus the baby enters the world protected, as far as antibodies can protect, against the same diseases as its mother.

A strong case can therefore be made for immunizing all women contemplating marriage against the infectious diseases prevalent in the community. Such a programme would be best undertaken during the engagement period.

How long do these antibodies survive?

Generally speaking Ig G antibodies have a half life of about 30 days. At this rate of disappearance there will be a negligible level of antibody concentration at about six or seven months of age. From this an important point emerges. Active immunization should be given from say the fifth or sixth month of age. To attempt active immunization before the third month is to run the risk of inhibition by the passively acquired antibody. Until the baby is actively immunized, that is until the fifth or sixth month, more than ordinary care should be taken to prevent contact with infectious diseases particularly whooping cough, diphtheria and measles.

Vaccination in childhood

To vaccinate or not to vaccinate is a clinical problem which in some cases may be difficult to solve. Each case would require to be considered on its own merits. Here only certain general principles concerning vaccination in childhood will be mentioned.

(1) Only vaccines from a reliable source should be used and the manufacturer's enclosure should be carefully studied in all cases.

(2) Vaccination should only be performed on healthy subjects. If there is a suspicion that the child is incubating an infection, vaccination should be postponed.

(3) Because of the numerous infections to which a child is susceptible the question of which vaccine should get priority arises. Special circumstances may dictate what action is to be taken. In normal circumstances, however, this problem has been largely solved by the availability of triple vaccine which protects against diphtheria, whooping cough and tetanus. With this combined vaccine, oral vaccine against poliomyelitis may be given. Generally speaking, the combined vaccine plus the oral vaccine against poliomyelitis should be given during the second six months of life.

(4) Should there be any untoward reaction with the combined vaccine the procedure may be continued with suitable individual vaccines.

IMMUNITY IN SPECIFIC DISEASES

Smallpox

The safest time for primary vaccination is between the first and the fourth year of life. This advice would have to be modified in countries where smallpox is epidemic. In western countries, however, postponing smallpox vaccination until the fourth year allows time for other, more urgent vaccinations to be carried out. Persons with dermatitis, whether adults or babies, should not be vaccinated until the dermatitis is completely cured, and, unless the risk is great, it is wise to postpone the vaccination of pregnant women. The virus has not been known to cause foetal deformities but occasional cases of generalized vaccinia of the foetus have been reported.

Vaccine

The material used for smallpox vaccination is live attenuated virus. Calves are the most commonly used source of the vaccine but it has been prepared from other sources as well. Some five or six days after the calf is vaccinated the vaccinial eruption appears. The animal is killed and the material in the eruption carefully collected and treated with phenol or some other antimicrobial agent for the purpose of reducing any contaminating organisms. Glycerol is then added to a concentration of about 50 per cent, the vaccine is then assayed, controlled and stored at −10 to −20°C. In some methods of production the vaccine is lyophilized. Such dried vaccine is stable for some years and offers great advantages in developing countries where smallpox is still a real problem.

Complications

Generalized vaccinia is probably the most important complication of smallpox vaccination at the present time. Should it occur the event ought to be reported to the manufacturers of the vaccine. For this, and other skin complications (eczema vaccinatum and vaccinia gangrenosa) anti-vaccinial gamma globulin may be used. Post-vaccinial encephalitis is an uncommon complication and occurs more frequently in adults being vaccinated for the first time. I myself, had it. Good results have been reported from the Netherlands on the use of anti-vaccinial gamma globulin in the solution of this problem.

Contra-indications to smallpox vaccination

(1) Any existing disease, especially skin disease, disease for which corticosteroid therapy is being given, and agammaglobulinaemia.

(2) History of recent exposure to infectious disease.

(3) Pregnancy.

Poliomyelitis

The almost complete conquest of poliomyelitis in several countries is the greatest triumph of immunology in recent years. Two kinds of vaccine are available–the Salk-type, which is inactivated and which stimulates the production of circulating antibodies; these antibodies attack the invaders during the viraemia stage of the disease and thus prevent involvement of the nervous system. The other kind of vaccine is the Sabin-type. This contains living attenuated viruses which become established in the intestinal wall where they multiply. Here they produce not only circulating antibodies but also a local immunity in the intestinal wall which prevents infection by virulent forms.

The attenuated vaccine has become the most popular. In addition to the advantage already stated, it is easy and inexpensive to administer. Sometimes, however, it may not work, and rarely it causes paralysis. The killed vaccine is effective but probably not as effective as the attenuated one. It is safe, or it ought to be.

Measles

The decline in the frequency and severity of measles in developed

106

countries such as Great Britain and the United States of America is likely to obscure the fact that it is still a very serious problem in less developed countries where it is not only more frequent but often so severe that it carries a mortality rate of up to 25 per cent.

For many years immunity or partial immunity could be conveyed by the intramuscular injection of (a) serum obtained from immune persons, (b) immune globulin extracted from human placenta, (c) gamma globulin obtained from human serum. The object in using these materials was, not to prevent the disease completely (except in weakly children) but to lessen its severity. In this way a permanent immunity usually resulted. The procedure, however, called for precise timing and this was often impossible.

The first strain of virus from which a vaccine was made was obtained from a patient named Edmonston and the virus is since known by that name. It was isolated by Enders and Peebles and passaged in such a way that two sub-strains were obtained. These are called A and B. From the Edmonston B, two further strains were evolved—these are known as the Beckenham 20 strain and the Schwartz strain. Both have been used extensively. The Schwartz strain is the more attenuated and therefore the safest, but the Beckenham strain may be the more effective in producing immunity. This illustrates a typical and recurring problem in vaccine production, balancing safety with potency.

A vaccine consisting of dead viruses was also developed but clinical trials proved that it was inadequate. It may, however, be used as an initial injection, to be followed in about one month by the live vaccine. In this way the incidence and severity of untoward reactions to the live virus are reduced.

Complications such as encephalitis have been reported after the use of the live virus vaccine alone, but in view of the great number of persons to whom the vaccine has been given, the incidence is very low.

German measles (rubella)

For many years German measles was considered a trivial disease; it was even considered as something of a joke. When Gregg discovered that the disease, when it occurred in pregnancy, could lead to abnormalities in the foetus (cateract, deafness, congenital heart disease and mental retardation) it took on a more sinister aspect. When it was discovered that it could occur without a rash and that even in this subclinical form it could lead to foetal abnormalities, it became more sinister still.

How great is the danger of foetal deformity?

Estimates vary. Originally it was stated to be 100 per cent in the first trimester and 75 per cent for pregnancy as a whole. Later estimates reduced the first figure to 10 per cent, but this may well be an underestimation. The true figure will probably never be known.

Protection

Gamma globulin given immediately after exposure seems to offer some protection but the whole idea of this approach is defective because a pregnant woman is unlikely to know exactly *when* or even *if* she has been exposed. In 1966 a live vaccine was introduced which seems to be satisfactory as far as producing immunity is concerned.

Who should be vaccinated?

A peculiar problem arises here. A high percentage of those vaccinated excrete the virus in the nasopharynx and thus may infect pregnant women; there is no reason to believe that this virus is harmless to the foetus. It should *not* be given to women who are, or who may be, or who may in the near future become, pregnant. What is required, therefore, is a vaccine which while being effective, does not render the vaccinated person infective to others. There is evidence that this has now been achieved by Meenan and colleagues using attenuated rubella virus of the Plotkin strain.

Mumps

Although mumps can on occasions be a severe infection, it is usually a trivial one. This doubtlessly explains why attempts to produce a vaccine have not been very active. Nevertheless, a vaccine is now available and so far it seems to be free from side effect. Its potency is adequate in that it induces antibodies in more than 95 per cent of cases. An advantage is that the injected virus is not transmitted to the unvaccinated, a problem that existed with rubella. Recently there has been a suggestion that mumps in a pregnant woman may affect the foetus. If this suggestion proves founded then there is a strong case for vaccinating women before they become pregnant.

Influenza

Two great difficulties arise in regard to the problem of influenza vaccination. Firstly, the disease may be caused by one of a number of antigenically distinct viruses. Therefore one cannot be sure which particular strain should be incorporated in the vaccine. Secondly, even if the correct strain is used, the immunity produced is short-lived. To be effective, therefore, the correct vaccine has to be given at the correct time and both of these criteria are hardly likely to be satisfied. If they are satisfied, however, an adequate degree of immunity is conveyed in a reasonable proportion of cases. There is obviously need for improvement here.

Common Cold

It has been estimated that about 25 per cent of the patients consulting general practitioners do so because of respiratory troubles and that, of these, about 33 per cent have colds. This says nothing about the number of people who never take a cold to a doctor. The common cold, therefore, though a trivial disease, is of great economic importance.

Colds may be caused by a great number of different viruses belonging to the groups of myxovirus, adenovirus, and picornavirus. Altogether there are about 100 serologically distinct types. There is little or no cross-reacting antibody produced when one of these types is used as a vaccine and therein lies the difficulty of producing an effective product. If it is discovered, however, that only a few of these virus types are responsible for the bulk of the epidemics, then the problem will be lessened.

Yellow Fever

A satisfactory live virus vaccine is available which gives protection for several years. As the virus is cultured in chick embryo it may cause severe reactions in those hypersensitive to eggs.

Rabies

A consideration of the sources of rabies suggests the people to whom protection should be given. Carnivores of various kinds are well known, but in some countries polecats, skunks, mongooses, meerkats, bats and monkeys have been incriminated. Active immunization is, therefore, recommended for laboratory workers, veterinarians, health inspectors and others whose work places them at risk.

The original material of Pasteur which consisted of a suspension of dried spinal cord of infected animals is no longer used because of the dangers involved. So perhaps Bernard Shaw had a point. Instead, the vaccines of Fermi, Semple, Hempt and others are now used in various parts of the world.

Typhus fever

Typhus is another example of a disease which has been controlled in recent years but for this credit must go, not to immunization, but to DDT and antibiotics. A living vaccine containing R. Prowazeki is available but it has not yet been properly proven. With the decreasing effectiveness of DDT and antibiotics the time may soon come when it will be.

Infective hepatitis

As the virus has not been isolated there is no vaccine available. Human gamma globulin has been recommended for those exposed to the disease but its value is questionable. A safe and effective means of active immunization is urgently required for this disease.

Homologous serum jaundice

As with infective hepatitis, the virus has not been isolated—hence there is no vaccine available. Human gamma globulin has been suggested as a means of passive immunization but its value is doubtful. It might, however, be given with advantage to selected recipients of blood and serum transfusions, especially in those areas where there is a high incidence of the disease.

Diphtheria

Diphtheria vaccination is often combined with vaccination against pertussis and tetanus. This is called the triple vaccine (DTP/Vac). Sometimes oral poliomyelitis is given at the same time. Here, however, each will be considered separately.

Active immunization

A variety of products are available for active immunization against diphtheria, so many, in fact, that there may be confusion. The following is suggested. For children under five years of age, purified toxoid aluminium phosphate (PTAP) in 0·5 ml doses should be given for primary immunization. The vaccine is prepared by adsorbing purified toxoid on aluminium phosphate which acts as an adjuvant. The first dose is given at about six months of age; this is followed by a second dose after one month, and this, by a third dose after six months. Booster doses may then be given on occasions of special risk or on entry to school.

For children between the ages of five and ten years of age, the same material may be used but the initial dose should be reduced to 0·2 ml.

For all those over ten years of age, the use of toxoid antitoxin floccules is preferred because it is less likely to cause unpleasant reactions. The dose is 0·5 ml, three times at monthly intervals. In this age group, only those who give a positive Schick test should be vaccinated.

Passive immunization

Passive immunization is achieved by the use of diphtheria antitoxin, a product usually derived from horses. It is used for both contacts and cases. Contacts may be given 1,000 to 2,000 units subcutaneously or intramuscularly. Immediate immunity is conferred but it is of short duration—hence, after three or four weeks, active immunization, as described above, should be instituted.

Because the material injected is derived from horse serum there is a risk of serum reactions. Although this risk is not as great as previously, certain precautions should be taken. The patient or the patient's parents should be questioned about any previous injections of horse serum, if there is doubt an intradermal injection using 0·1 ml of a 1 in 10 dilution of the antiserum should be given as a test. In all cases, adrenaline and coramine should be at hand.

Desensitization

If there is a reaction to the test dose then desensitization may be attempted. A 1 in 10 dilution of the antiserum is used. This special dilution is available commercially, if required; 0·1 ml is given subcutaneously. If there is no reaction after half an hour, 0·2 ml is given. After another half hour, if there is no reaction, 0·4 ml is given. And so on, every half hour, if there is no reaction the previous dose is doubled until eight doses have been given.

Pertussis

Pertussis is a serious disease in young babies and generally, the younger the baby the more serious it is. For this reason it was formerly advised that vaccination against pertussis be started at two months of age or even earlier. More recently it has been suggested that a better and more lasting immunity is obtained if vaccination is deferred until about six months of age. Until this age reliance is placed on strict protection of the baby against infection. This may not be an easy task in certain areas due to over-crowding and especially if there is a high incidence of pertussis. The practitioner therefore must decide each case on its own particular circumstances.

The vaccine consists of dead Bordetella pertussis organisms; its

111

potency and safety are now well established; 0·5 ml is given subcutaneously at four week or preferably six week intervals. A booster dose may be given twelve months later and at time of special risk.

In practice it is far more convenient for patient, doctor and parent if the combined vaccine (DTP/Vac) is used, and it may be used as a routine, but in special circumstances separate vaccination is indicated.

Tetanus

Far too many people die of tetanus. Despite the availability of an effective vaccine, it is said that tetanus causes 50,000 deaths each year—and horrible deaths they must be. Active immunization is particularly indicated in soldiers, veterinarians and those engaged in agricultural work. Though an enthusiastic gardener, I would not dream of working in my garden without the protection of tetanus toxoid. My determination in this matter was reinforced not long ago when my next door neighbour told me over the garden fence that he had a stiff jaw. He had tetanus, and he very nearly died.

The material used is formol-toxoid. It is prepared by heating the toxin in the presence of formalin until it is no longer toxic. One ml followed by another in eight weeks, followed by a third in six months gives good immunity, but in special cases the intervals may be shortened. A booster dose of 0·5 ml may be given after five years.

Recently, tetanus vaccine purified toxoid aluminium phosphate BP, has become available. This adsorbed toxoid has definite advantages over the former product. There is a better antibody response and by its use active-passive immunization (ATS) can be given immediately to those patients who receive such wounds as might result in tetanus. With the original product, the administration of ATS interferes with the antigen.

Probably every case of tetanus can be prevented. To achieve this there must be universal immunization at an early age and booster injections every four or five years thereafter. Such a programme will also solve the problem of whether to give or to withhold ATS (horse serum) in patients with minor wounds.

Passive immunization

Tetanus antiserum (ATS) is available for those specially exposed to risk, that is, those with wounds which might lead to tetanus. The antiserum is often prepared in horses—hence, if it is used, the same principles (and risks) as in the use of diphtheria antiserum apply here also.

In recent years, human tetanus immune globulin has become

available. It is said to be remarkably effective in conferring passive immunity and it is, of course, free from the dangers associated with the injection of foreign serum.

Tuberculosis

A live vaccine which consists of an attenuated bovine strain of mycobacterium tuberculosis is used. This organism was first introduced by Calmette and Guerin in 1921 and is commonly known as BCG (Bacille Calmette-Guerin). It is administered through multiple punctures in the skin which are conveniently made by means of the Heaf instrument.

The object of BCG vaccination is to produce, not antibodies, but a state of delayed hypersensitivity which, under natural conditions, is produced by primary tuberculosis. As tuberculin positive persons may have severe reactions to this vaccine, the Mantoux test should first be done and only those giving a negative result should be vaccinated. Infants are often presumed to be Mantoux negative and this seems to be a reasonable presumption.

The vaccine is effective but there is some disagreement about how effective it is. In a disease like tuberculosis this is obviously a very difficult point to assess. There is probably room for improvement.

Leprosy

As mycobacterium leprae, the organism which causes leprosy, has never been cultured *in vitro*, there is no specific vaccine available. In 1939, however, Fernandes noticed that a large proportion of lepromin-negative children became lepromin-positive after vaccination with BCG. This suggested to Fernandes that BCG might confer immunity to leprosy. Since that time extensive trials have been carried out to test the suggestion but the results were equivocal. Still, better BCG than nothing.

Syphilis

The immunological reactions to the spirochaete of syphilis have always been baffling. It is known that the antibody detected by the treponemal immobilization test kills the organism in the presence of complement and it is, therefore, reasonable to think that it is protective. There is, in addition, a cellular reaction to infection by the spirochaete which also seems to be protective. Vaccination, therefore, seems feasible. Yet vaccines, consisting of dead organisms, have been tried and found wanting.

Spirochaetes have been rendered non-pathogenic by the use of γ

radiation. Such organisms still retain their antigenicity and are being further investigated with vaccine production in view. Also, Treponema cuniculi, an organism which causes venereal disease in rabbits, but which is capable of producing cross-reacting antibodies against Treponema pallidum, is a possible source of vaccine.

Peculiar problems

Two peculiar problems arise in connection with vaccination against syphilis. If the vaccine causes a positive Wasserman reaction, which it may well do, then the diagnosis of syphilis will be a more difficult task than it is at present. As the control of syphilis depends upon prompt diagnosis and treatment, anything which militates against diagnosis will also militate against control. What is needed, therefore, is a vaccine which will confer immunity but which will not, at the same time, cause false positive serological reactions for syphilis. That seems a tall order.

The other problem is that of who precisely should be vaccinated. It could hardly be made compulsory but if it is not, who is going to volunteer for it? Furthermore, what view will the Church and civil authorities take towards a vaccine which is almost certain to be accused of being an inducement to sin?

Typhoid fever

Although vaccination against typhoid fever has been in use for more than 50 years, we are still in doubt about its effectiveness. The great difficulty is that it is almost impossible to assess the value of a vaccine when other factors which militate against the disease are operating at the same time. In typhoid fever there is another difficulty in that the identical disease cannot be conveyed to laboratory animals. Hence this means of assessing potency is not possible. Even the method of making and administering the vaccine has been questioned and it has been suggested that the intradermal route gives a better antibody response than the subcutaneous route.

Field trials strongly suggest that vaccines are effective, though not completely effective. Furthermore, some vaccines are more effective than others. No doubt vaccines prepared from local strains of the organism are more effective than those imported from elsewhere.

The vaccine

The traditional material consists of heat-killed phenolized typhoid and paratyphoid organisms (TAB). The paratyphoid organisms seem to have been included for good measure. They contribute to the pain of the injection but there is no evidence that they are effective in preventing paratyphoid fever.

In view of the reservations concerning its effectiveness, the vaccine should be given to those at risk, but it must be stressed that this should not lead to complacency in regard to the other preventive measures in common use against typhoid fever. There is still no substitute for cleanliness. The intradermal method of administration is growing in popularity, probably because it is more comfortable for the patient.

Cholera

A heat-killed vaccine containing smooth strains of the two main types of V. Cholerae is available. Sometimes cholera vaccine is combined with typhoid vaccine (TABC). Most of what has been said about typhoid vaccine applies also to cholera vaccine so there is obviously room for improvement.

Plague

A formalin-killed vaccine is available. Its value, however, is questionable. I myself had the vaccine when I was working with plague and I did not contract the disease. But other workers did, so again there is obviously need for improvement.

Test questions

CHAPTER 1

1   What is an antigen?
2   What are the conditions for antigenicity?
3   What is the usual chemical nature of an antigen?
4   Give two examples of carbohydrate antigens.
5   What is a toxoid?
6   What is Witebsky substance?
7   What is meant by Forssman antigens?
8   What is Ehrlich's principle of *horror autotoxicus*?
9   What is a chimera?
10   What do chimeras teach us about immunology?
11   What is meant by the critical point of Medawar?
12   What is a hapten?
13   What is the Australian antigen?
14   What is an adjuvant?

CHAPTER 2

1   What is an antibody?
2   What is the chemical nature of an antibody?
3   What is meant by gamma globulin?
4   What is meant by the 'naturally occurring antibodies'?
5   Name the naturally occurring iso-antibodies.
6   What is the significance of anti-C?
7   What is the origin of the naturally occurring iso-antibodies?
8   What is meant by antibody specificity?
9   What is a cross-reaction?
10   What is meant by complete and incomplete antibodies?
11   What is meant by cold and warm antibodies?
12   What is an autoantibody?
13   How is the strength of an antiserum measured? Discuss.
14   What is complement?

116

CHAPTER 3

1 Compare the direct and indirect theories of antibody production.
2 Discuss Jerne's theory of antibody production.
3 Discuss the clonal selection theory of Burnet.
4 What is the lymphocyte receptor theory?
5 What is meant by 'lymphoid' tissue?
6 In what organs and tissues are antibodies produced?
7 By which cells are antibodies produced? Discuss.

CHAPTER 4

1 Draw a diagram showing the basic structure of an immunoglobulin molecule.
2 Name the symbols given to the heavy and light chains.
3 What is the effect of papain digestion of an immunoglobulin molecule?
4 What is Fab? Why is it so called?
5 What is the importance of placenta-crossing immunoglobulins?
6 What are Bence-Jones proteins?
7 Write a note on the allotypes of Ig G.
8 Write notes on Ig M, Ig A and Ig E.

CHAPTER 5

1 How are precipitin reactions demonstrated?
2 What is meant by immunoelectrophoresis?
3 How are agglutination reactions demonstrated?
4 What is an agglutination-inhibition test?
5 Discuss the importance of incomplete antibodies.
6 Describe the indirect Coombs test.
7 State the principle of the Wasserman reaction.
8 State the principle of the indirect Coons test.
9 Describe the Schultz-Dale reaction.

CHAPTER 6

1 Name the three well-defined immunological responses.
2 Write a note on Type 1 responses.
3 Describe the difference between primary and secondary antigenic stimulation.

4   What is meant by natural immunity?
5   By what age does a baby produce its own antibodies?
6   What is meant by 'allergen'?
7   What is 'reagin' type antibody?
8   Describe the pathogenesis of immediate hypersensitivity.
9   Name the active substances liberated in immediate hypersensitivity.
10   What is the Prausnitz-Kustner reaction?
11   How was delayed hypersensitivity discovered?
12   Discuss the role of the thymus gland in immunology.

CHAPTER 7

1   Discuss 'agammaglobulinaemia'.
2   What is the normal concentration of Ig G in the serum?
3   Discuss the treatment for hypogammaglobulinaemia.
4   What is meant by the Swiss type of agammaglobulinaemia?
5   How does disease of the thymus gland throw light on immunological processes?
6   How can a functional deficiency of the immunoglobulins be recognized?
7   Discuss myelomatosis.
8   Write a note on Waldenstrom's macroglobulinaemia.

CHAPTER 8

1   Name five familiar immediate hypersensitivity reactions.
2   Name two varieties of grass pollen which cause hay fever.
3   State how psychological factors may complicate the clinical diagnosis of immediate hypersensitivity reactions.
4   Describe the principles of the treatment of asthma.
5   How may penicillin hypersensitivity be acquired?
6   Describe the treatment of a hypersensitivity reaction due to penicillin.
7   Outline a routine for skin testing in cases of immediate hypersensitivity.
8   Write a note on desensitization.

CHAPTER 9

1   What features distinguish delayed from immediate hypersensitivity?

2   What is the tuberculin test?

3   Describe the microscopic appearance of the skin lesion in the tuberculin test.

4   Discuss the significance of delayed hypersensitivity in tuberculosis.

5   Discuss the significance of delayed hypersensitivity in diseases other than tuberculosis.

6   Discuss Type 1 immunological responses in homograft rejection.

7   Discuss Type 3 immunological responses in homograft rejection.

8   Discuss the evidence for a relationship between delayed hypersensitivity and malignant growth.

CHAPTER 10

1   What do you understand by 'allergy'.

2   Contrast immunity with hypersensitivity.

3   Classify 'allergy'.

4   What is the Arthus phenomenon? Discuss its pathogenesis.

5   Contrast the Arthus phenomenon with classical immediate hypersensitivity.

6   What is anaphylaxis? Discuss its pathogenesis.

7   What is serum sickness? Discuss its pathogenesis.

8   Serum sickness occurs about a week after antigenic stimulation, yet it is an example of immediate hypersensitivity. Explain.

9   What are the advantages and disadvantages of using therapeutic antisera prepared in human beings?

10   What is meant by 'Farmer's lung'? Discuss its aetiology.

11   What organisms abound in mouldy hay?

CHAPTER 11

1   Name the important blood group systems. In what ways are they important?

2   How are the ABO blood groups determined in the laboratory?

3   What is Landsteiner's rule?

4   Discuss the evidence for the existence of anti-C.

5   What is the clinical significance of anti-C?

6   How is group A_1 distinguished from group A_2?

7   What is the importance of the A_2 antigen?

8   How was the Rh blood group system discovered?

9 In what way did the discovery of anti-rh′ and anti-rh″ extend our knowledge of the Rh blood group system.

10 What is meant by Rh?

11 What is the importance of the Rh variants?

12 Contrast the two Rh nomenclatures in current use.

13 Describe the serological reactions given by group CDE and group cde.

14 Describe the serological reactions given by group Rh_z and group rh.

15 What is the main practical application of the MN blood group system?

16 Name the eight groups of blood stocked by blood banks.

CHAPTER 12

1 State Rule 1 and Rule 2 of blood transfusion.

2 How are these rules satisfied?

3 Why is it necessary to group *and* cross-match in blood transfusion?

4 If a transfusion is required for a newborn baby, it is usual to cross-match using the mother's serum. Why?

5 Why are the mother's red cells always compatible with the baby's serum?

6 What is meant by high titre and low titre group O blood?

7 Discuss the concept of 'Universal' donors and recipients.

8 How may a latent haemolytic reaction be brought to light?

9 What is the connection between dextran (and other such products) and the cross-matching test?

10 Discuss the difficulties in cross-matching in cases of auto-allergic haemolytic anaemia.

11 How do haemolytic transfusion reactions arise?

12 Describe the clinical features of a haemolytic transfusion reaction.

13 What are the first steps in the management of a haemolytic transfusion reaction?

14 Discuss immunological reactions, other than haemolytic reactions, following blood transfusion.

CHAPTER 13

1 What is meant by a homospecific and a heterospecific pregnancy?

2   Discuss the difficulties in the diagnosis of **ABO** haemolytic disease.

3   In view of these difficulties, how should a suspected case be managed?

4   Which of the Rh factors is the most important as a cause of Rh disease?

5   In what ways may a woman become immunized to the Rh factor?

6   What percentage of marriages in a European community are marriages between Rh negative women and Rh positive men?

7   What bearing has the zygosity of the father on the incidence of Rh disease?

8   How does the materno-foetal ABO situation affect the incidence of Rh disease?

9   Why is the firstborn so seldom affected with Rh disease?

10   Why is Rh disease a lesser problem in Negroes than in people of European descent?

11   Discuss the pathogenesis of ABO haemolytic disease.

12   Discuss the pathogenesis of Rh haemolytic disease.

13   What are the objects of antenatal immunological care? How are these objects achieved?

CHAPTER 14

1   Discuss the circumstances in which domestic antigens may become antigenically active.

2   Write a note on autoallergic haemolytic anaemia of the warm type.

3   Write a note on autoallergic haemolytic anaemia of the cold type.

4   Discuss the role of autoantibodies in the pathogenesis of Hashimoto's disease.

5   Discuss the evidence of delayed hypersensitivity in the aetiology of Hashimoto's disease.

6   Discuss the evidence of an immunological basis for rheumatoid arthritis.

7   State the points in favour of lupus erythematosus being an autoallergic disease.

8   Describe the autoantibodies which have been discovered in cases of pernicious anaemia.

9   Discuss ulcerative colitis as an autoallergic disease.

CHAPTER 15

1 For which diseases are there reasonably reliable serological tests available for diagnosis?
2 What is the all-important point to be noted when interpreting the results of serological tests?
3 Discuss the Widal test for typhoid fever.
4 Discuss the serological diagnosis of brucella infection.
5 Discuss the gonococcal complement-fixation test.
6 What antibodies occur in the serum in cases of glandular fever?
7 Discuss the serological diagnosis of syphilis.
8 Discuss the serological diagnosis of amoebiasis.
9 Describe the LE cell. What is its significance?
10 Discuss the serological tests which are of value in the diagnosis of rheumatoid arthritis.
11 Compare rheumatoid arthritis with lupus erythematosus.
12 What antibodies occur in the serum in cases of Hashimoto's disease?
13 Name five skin tests which depend on a delayed hypersensitivity response.
14 Describe the Kveim test for sarcoidosis.
15 Write a note on the Schick test.

CHAPTER 16

1 Against which diseases are there reasonably safe and effective vaccines available?
2 Against which disease is there urgent need for a safe and reliable vaccine?
3 What are the difficulties in assessing the value of a vaccine?
4 What materials are commonly used for vaccination?
5 Why should vaccination schedules be revised from time to time?
6 At approximately what age should a baby be vaccinated? Why?
7 Outline the method by which smallpox vaccine is prepared.
8 What are the complications of smallpox vaccination?
9 Write a note on poliomyelitis vaccines.
10 Discuss the means available for preventing measles.
11 What are the problems of rubella vaccination?
12 What are the difficulties in producing effective vaccines against influenza and the common cold?

13   Discuss vaccination against diphtheria.
14   Write a note on the importance of tetanus vaccination.
15   What materials are available for tetanus vaccination?
16   Discuss vaccination against tuberculosis and leprosy.
17   Discuss vaccination against typhoid fever and cholera.

References

Darwin, C. (1856). *Origin of the Species by Means of Natural Selection*, London, John Murray

Gell, P. G. H. and Coombs, R. R. A. (1963). *Clinical Aspects of Immunology*, Oxford, Blackwell Scientific Publications.

Jenner, E. (1800). *An Enquiry into the Causes and Effects of Variola Vaccinae*, London, Sampson Low

Jerne, U. K. (1955). "The Natural Selection Theory of Antibody Formation." *Proc. Nat. Acad. Sci.* **41**, 849.

Mitchnikoff, E. (1903). *The Nature of Man*, London, Heinemann Ltd.

— (1904). *Old Age.*

— (1905). *Immunity to Infectious Diseases*, Cambridge University Press.

— (1906). *Some Observations on Soured Milk.*

Payling Wright, G. (1954). *An Introduction to Pathology*, London, Longmans Green and Co Ltd.

Shaw, G. B. (1906). *The Doctor's Dilemma*, London, Constable and Co. Ltd.

Wade, H. (1908). *Journal of Path. and Bact.* **12**, 384.

Index